MIND BOOSTERS

PREVIOUS PUBLICATIONS BY DR. RAY SAHELIAN, M.D.

The Common Cold Cure (with Victoria Dolby Toews)

The Stevia Cookbook: Cooking with Nature's Calorie-Free Sweetener (with Donna Gates)

All About Glucosamine and Chondroitin

Kava: The Miracle Antianxiety Herb (available from St. Martin's Press)

Creatine: Nature's Muscle Builder (with Dave Tuttle)

All About CoQ10

See *www.raysahelian.com* for updates
on natural supplements and mind boosters.

MIND BOOSTERS

A Guide to Natural Supplements That Enhance Your Mind, Memory, and Mood

RAY SAHELIAN, M.D.

ST. MARTIN'S GRIFFIN
NEW YORK

MIND BOOSTERS: A GUIDE TO NATURAL SUPPLEMENTS THAT ENHANCE YOUR MIND, MEMORY, AND MOOD.

Figures 3.2, 3.4, and 3.5 reprinted with permission from M.A. Schmidt, *Smart Fats: How Dietary Fats and Oils Affect Mental, Physical, and Emotional Intelligence*, (Berkeley, Calif.: Frog Ltd., 1997).

www.stmartins.com

Book design by Casey Hampton

ISBN 0-312-19584-2

10 9 8 7 6

A NOTE TO READERS

This book is for informational purposes only. Readers are advised to consult a trained medical professional before acting on any of the information in this book. The fact that a particular nutrient, herb, or supplement is discussed in the book in connection with an illness or condition does not necessarily mean that it is safe and appropriate for everyone or that the author or publisher recommends its use for that illness or condition.

CONTENTS

PART IV: A PRACTICAL GUIDE TO MIND-BOOSTING SUPPLEMENTS

PART V: STAYING SMART AFTER SCHOOL

PART VI: NATURAL PRESCRIPTIONS FOR DEPRESSION, VISION ENHANCEMENT, ALZHEIMER'S, AND PARKINSON'S DISEASE

ACKNOWLEDGMENTS

Lise Alschuler, N.D., is Chair of the Botanical Medicine Department at Bastyr University in Seattle, Washington.

David Benton, Ph.D., is Professor of Psychology at the University of Wales in Swansea. He researches the influence of B vitamins on mood and cognition.

Robert Clarke, Ph.D., from the Clinical Trial Service Unit at Radcliffe Infirmary in Oxford, England, researches the influence of homocysteine on the brain.

Craig Cooney, Ph.D., Research Assistant Professor at University of Arkansas for Medical Sciences, Little Rock, Arkansas, is an expert on methyl donors.

Tom Hamazaki, M.D., Ph.D., is at the Department of Internal Medicine, Toyama Medical and Pharmaceutical University, in Toyama, Japan. He studies the effect of fish oils on stress and hostility.

Joseph R. Hibbeln, M.D., is Chief of the Outpatient Clinic, Laboratory of Membrane Biochemistry and Biophysics, National Institute on Alcohol Abuse and Alcoholism, in Rockville, Maryland. Dr. Hibbeln is an expert in omega-3 fatty acids.

Lloyd Horrocks, Ph. D., is professor emeritus of medical biochemistry at Ohio State University, Columbus, Ohio, and an expert in fatty acids.

Burton J. Litman, Ph.D., at the Laboratory of Membrane Biochemistry and Biophysics, at the National Institutes of Health in Rockville, Maryland, is an expert in the biochemistry of vision.

Mark Mattson, Ph.D., is Professor of Anatomy and Neurobiology at the University of Kentucky Sanders-Brown Center on Aging in Lexington, Kentucky. He studies the effect of caloric restriction on the course of neurodegenerative conditions.

Kilmer McCully, M.D., from Pathological Services at Veterans Affairs Medical Center, in Providence, Rhode Island, is a pioneer in homocysteine research.

Lucilla Parnetti, M.D., Ph.D., at the Institute of Nervous and Mental Diseases, Perugia University in Perugia, Italy, is an expert on Alzheimer's disease.

Malcolm Peet, M.D., is at the Department of Psychiatry, Northern General Hospital, in Sheffield, England. He studies the influence of fish oils on schizophrenia.

Vittorio Porciatti, Ph.D., at the Institute of Neurophysiology in Pisa, Italy, has studied the effects of CDP-choline on vision.

Helga Refsum, M.D., from Bergen University in Norway, researches the role of homocysteine in Alzheimer's disease.

Norman Salem Jr., Ph.D., is Acting Scientific Director at the National Institute on Alcohol Abuse and Alcoholism in Rockville, Maryland, and Chief, Laboratory of Membrane Biochemistry and Biophysics, at the National Institutes of Health. Dr. Salem is an expert in omega-3 fatty acids.

Artemis P. Simopoulos, M.D., President for the Center for Genetics, Nutrition and Health in Washington, D.C., is an expert on fatty acids.

Andrew L. Stoll, M.D., is at the Psychopharmacology Unit, Brigham and Women's School, Department of Psychiatry, Harvard Medical School. He studies the effects of fish oils on bipolar disorders.

Owen Wolkowitz, M.D., from the Department of Psychiatry at the

University of San Francisco, studies the influence of hormones on mood and memory.

Shlomo Yehuda, Ph.D., from the Department of Psychology, Bar Ilan University, Ramat Gan, in Israel, studies the influence of polyunsaturated fatty acids on brain cells.

Steven H. Zeisel, M.D., Ph.D., is Professor and Chairman, Department of Nutrition, University of North Carolina at Chapel Hill, North Carolina, and one of the world's leading experts on choline and phospholipids.

My thanks also to the following individuals for the information they provided: Steven Bock, M.D.; David P. Crass, M.D.; Thomas Crook, Ph.D.; Subhuti Dharmananda, Ph.D.; Barry Elson, M.D.; Paul Frankl, Ph.D.; Terry Grossman, M.D.; Abram Hoffer, Ph.D., M.D.; Joseph P. Horrigan, M.D.; David Horrobin, DPhil (Stirling, UK), Dharma Singh Khalsa, M.D.; David Kyle, Ph.D.; Danise Lehrer, O.M.D.; Jay L. Lombard, D.O.; Fred Madsen, Ph.D.; Lester Packer, Ph.D.; Mason Panetti; Ascanio Polimeni, M.D. (Rome, Italy); Jo Robinson, Michael Schmidt, Shailinder Sodhi, N.D.; Karlis Ullis, M.D.; Roy Upton, Benita von Klingspor, and Byron Weston, M.D.

INTRODUCTION

Over the past few years, dozens of new natural supplements have been introduced that promise to enhance mental function. It may be quite daunting for you to walk into a vitamin store and see shelves and shelves of products that claim to improve memory, intelligence, mood, sex drive, vision, and mental performance. Many of these products are also promoted as playing a positive role in preventing or treating certain psychiatric and neurological disorders. How do you determine which of these supplements is appropriate for you? And how do you decide how much to take, in what combinations, how often, and for how long? The whole process is admittedly complicated. Even health-care practitioners experienced in nutritional therapy can't make complete sense of it all.

I have always been fascinated by how nutrition affects the mind. This interest motivated me to seek an undergraduate degree in nutrition science. I then attended Thomas Jefferson Medical School in Philadelphia, and later completed a three-year residency in family practice. Over the past two decades I have reviewed thousands of published articles on nutrients that have an influence on brain health; and have also supervised patients interested in improving their mental performance. I have discovered that the benefits of nutrients are often quick and remarkable, and in many cases equivalent or superior to those obtained by pharmaceutical drugs. There is no doubt that many of these brain supplements enhance quality of life. My goal in writing this book has been to gather the relevant published and clinical information regarding the role of dietary supplements on the mind, properly categorize it, and present it in a straightforward and practical way that can help consumers and health-care practitioners alike.

The medical community has not adequately investigated the use of natural supplements for the purposes of mental enhancement or for the therapy of neurological and psychiatric disorders. My hope is that the information presented in *Mind Boosters: A Guide to Natural Supplements that Enhance Your Mind, Memory, and Mood* will help patients improve their mental capacities in a safe and natural way. It is also my wish that more physicians become aware of these supplements and prescribe them to their patients, thus lessening reliance on pharmaceutical drugs. If your health-care practitioner is not familiar with any of these supplements, recommend that he or she review this book.

An amazing aspect of the brain is its ability to improve its own performance. A computer certainly can't improve its hardware or software on its own. By using our intellect to make the right choices, we can make ourselves even smarter. By cautiously and intelligently taking advantage of the variety of natural supplements currently at our disposal, we can help our brains function better, faster, and more efficiently—as well as treat many brain disorders in a more natural way. It is now also possible to take advantage of the growing scientific knowledge regarding brain nutrition to help keep our brains young as long as possible.

I do not sell or endorse supplements. In the following chapters, you will find a discussion not only of the benefits of these nutrients, but also their shortcomings. I will also inform you on how not to waste your hard-earned dollars on nutrients that either don't work well, or could easily be obtained from your diet.

The premise of this book is that you already have tried, or are currently trying, many of the non-pill approaches to improving your memory and mind. A brief discussion on simple non-pill steps to a better brain is presented in Part III. But perhaps you are now searching for additional avenues to enhance your mental performance. The comprehensive and practical information presented in *Mind Boosters* will help you attain your goal.

PART I

Using Your Brain to Boost Your Mind

ONE

The Born-Again Brain

We live in an age when we are constantly barraged by information from dozens of television channels, daily newspapers, weekly and monthly magazines, faxes, e-mails, and the endless data posted on the Internet. Even the young and healthy are overwhelmed trying to keep up with this accelerated rate of information overload. The modern world seems to be requiring too much effort from our mental abilities.

Fortunately, science continues to discover ways to enhance the mind's performance. Enough research evidence has now been accumulated to give scientists a detailed picture of how the brain's intricate machinery works. This understanding makes it easier for us to use the variety of supplements currently available to provide the nutritional, neurochemical, and hormonal substances necessary for the brain's optimal functioning. Enhancing one's mind no longer depends on guesswork. Doctors now can manipulate the brain with a good deal of certainty in order to increase intelligence and mental productivity, and to help treat several mental disorders that previously required the exclusive use of pharmaceutical drugs. I propose that the intelligent use of natural supplements can improve our mind, memory, and mood, and help us better adapt to this information onslaught.

Supplements are also beneficial in additional situations. Many individuals report a fear of losing their mental abilities as they get older. Some are afraid of getting Alzheimer's disease or Parkinson's disease, especially if they have parents or relatives with these conditions. But these diseases affect only a small portion of the population compared to those who have a "normal" loss of brain function with aging. In fact, there's even a term coined for "normal" brain aging: it's called ARCD.

AGE-RELATED COGNITIVE DECLINE (ARCD)

Also known as "age-associated memory impairment," ARCD is a term applied to individuals who experience age-related loss in cognition. The word *cognition* refers to mental activities such as thinking, memory, learning, and perception. Cognitive loss occurs to some degree in almost everybody. We lose our ability to easily remember telephone numbers and names, do mathematical calculations, and learn new concepts. However, some individuals experience a faster cognitive decline than most. This decline can be very frustrating, especially if a person wishes to continue working in an intellectually demanding career that requires fast thinking and a full memory capacity.

Is this decline in mental functioning inevitable, or are there steps we can take to slow down, stop, or even reverse this process? New scientific research indicates that there are nutritional therapies that can have a positive influence in improving mental function in middle and old age. These nutritional therapies are readily available over the counter. The research is accumulating so quickly that the difficulty lies in knowing how to best take practical advantage of this information.

Several medical conditions can also play a role in the decline of cognitive functioning. The most common include hypertension, atherosclerosis, and stroke. We must also recognize that, in older age groups, there are medicines prescribed for a variety of conditions that could have negative effects on brain health. Of course, cognitive decline also occurs as a consequence of neurological disorders such as Alzheimer's disease and Parkinson's disease.

Although the causes of ARCD are not fully understood, we know that it involves multiple changes in the brain. Thus, in order to treat ARCD effectively, several aspects of brain-cell health have to be addressed simultaneously.

WHAT CAN NATURAL SUPPLEMENTS DO FOR YOU?

Through many years of delving into the deep secrets of the brain, scientists have started to recognize that natural nutrients can improve

- Learning and memory
- Alertness and mental arousal
- Mood, energy, and vitality
- Speed of thinking and reaction time
- Verbal fluency and capacity to be humorous
- Concentration and focus
- Creativity and development of novel concepts
- Complex problem-solving abilities
- Sex drive and sexual enjoyment
- Vision, hearing, awareness, and sensory perception

Yes, it's true. Some of these supplements can even improve vision and hearing, senses that are intricately associated with awareness.

Many doctors are now beginning to recommend natural methods as therapies of cognitive impairment. Although natural substances can't yet completely replace the benefits of some pharmaceutical medicines in treating certain chronic neurological conditions, they can provide a number of advantages with a lower risk of side effects. The proper use of certain nutrients could potentially lessen the required dosage of pharmaceutical drugs.

There are skeptics, including doctors, who claim, "There's no such thing as a natural supplement that can improve brain function. It's all hype." Whenever I hear someone saying this, I immediately suspect that this person has little or no personal or professional experience with these supplements. Many studies have been published reporting the positive effects of nutrients, herbs, and hormones as they relate to improving brain function. Many of these natural supplements can even act as powerful antioxidants that may prevent or slow the degeneration of brain cells that almost invariably occurs with time.

However promising and persuasive the results of published studies, many people are not entirely convinced that mind "boosters" work until they take them themselves. Once you personally notice the enhancement in mood, memory, energy, thinking ability, and visual perception, you won't need the results of a double-blind study to be swayed that these natural pills really do work.

Having said this, I do wish to emphasize that the brain is an extremely complicated organ, and much remains unknown about its functions and nutritional requirements. In *Mind Boosters* I present to you, the intelligent reader, the latest information on natural supplements and how they affect the brain. It will then be up to you, in consultation with your health-care provider, to decide whether these supplements are appropriate for your unique circumstance.

There are at least two types of individuals (including both patients and physicians)—conservatives who want to wait until more information is published before taking a particular course of action, and optimists who don't mind taking supplements based on preliminary information. Where do you fit in?

PERSONALIZING YOUR MIND-BOOSTING REGIMEN

In this book I discuss and evaluate many nutrients, herbs, amino acids, and hormones. Then I take it a step further by providing you with an individualized regimen. This is based on your age group and your preference for nutrients, herbs, or hormones. In addition, I have provided step-by-step recommendations for which supplements to try first, and how you can combine them to achieve the best possible response. Keep in mind that these are just guidelines. Your requirements and responses may vary depending on your biochemical makeup.

It may take trial and error to find out which of the supplements discussed in this book are appropriate for you. Everyone is different, and you may not respond to a particular supplement that others find very helpful. Or, you could find one supplement that gives you a wonderful cognitive enhancement, while another person experiences a side effect and thinks it's a terrible pill. The dosage requirements could also vary significantly. Some individuals may require a large amount of a particular nutrient due to their body's lack of the proper enzymes to make this nutrient on its own. Another person could notice a positive effect from a tiny dosage.

THE IMPORTANCE OF MEDICAL SUPERVISION

The natural supplements discussed in this book are readily available over-the-counter, either in health-food stores, retail outlets, pharmacies, or through mail-order vitamin companies. I recommend that you consult with your health-care practitioner before you take any of these supplements. Many of these pills are very potent and could interact with medicines you may take, or they could influence the course of a previously existing medical condition. Some of them have significant side effects if misused. One can't assume that just because a supplement is available over the counter, that it is completely safe at any dose.

THE EXPERIENCE OF PATIENTS AND USERS

Mind Boosters includes the latest published studies regarding a wide range of supplements that influence the mind. Since research on some of these supplements is extremely limited, we have little practical information on how they affect the average person who takes them. In fact, some of these supplements have been introduced to the public with hardly any human trials having been performed. Moreover, little is known regarding the combination of two or more nutrients, hormones, or herbs.

In order to provide you with additional insights on what people really notice when they take these supplements, I have included brief case reports from actual users. Many of these are from my patients, and some are from interviews I conducted with individuals who regularly use natural brain boosters. Over the years, I have met many individuals who take brain supplements and I regularly keep in touch with them to discuss their experiences. I have included anecdotes in this book only when a number of users have reported similar experiences. For instance, I have reports from dozens of patients and individuals who notice visual enhancement from the hormone pregnenolone. Therefore, even though human trials regarding pregnenolone's effect on vision have not been published, I am convinced that this occurs.

I understand that including anecdotes may provoke criticism from the medical community. Science generally frowns upon anecdotal evidence, and for good reason: this type of information can sometimes be incomplete or even misleading. Nevertheless, until additional formal studies are available, anecdotes are a primary source of knowledge and can sometimes provide information not otherwise available.

THE EXPERIENCE OF CLINICIANS AND EXPERTS

I strongly believe that a physician with good observation skills can sometimes observe effects from nutrients or drugs that have been missed or overlooked in published studies. Thus, I have sometimes included reports from clinicians and experts who use nutrients and herbs in their practice. Scientific studies often lag years, decades, or sometimes hundreds of years behind clinical observations. For instance, St. John's wort has been recognized to improve mood by European doctors since the Middle Ages. Polynesians knew for centuries that kava reduces anxiety. Yet it wasn't until the 1990s that scientists finally acknowledged the clinical effects of these herbs.

THE AUTHOR'S EXPERIENCE

Before I write about supplements, or recommend them to patients, I try to find out for myself what effects they have on me. I often encounter positive and negative effects that have not been previously reported in the medical literature. For instance, I have observed that melatonin makes dreams more vivid. This effect had not been previously reported in the medical literature. I have also observed that a large intake of fish or flaxseed oils improves visual perception. Again, these observations have not been reported in the medical literature. In these two particular cases, I believe that my observations are accurate. Scientists often miss very obvious findings even in placebo-controlled, double-blind studies. This could be due to the inexperience of the researchers; not asking the right questions; not performing the right laboratory tests; misinterpreting the findings; the bias of the researchers; or poor statistical analyses. Furthermore, research methods are sometimes not able to recognize subtle changes or effects from medicines.

Over the past few years, I have experimented with almost all of the supplements discussed in this book, and have included accounts of some of my experiences. I believe these accounts will help you better understand the effects you may notice immediately if you take these supplements. Having experimented with several dozen natural supplements in varying dosages for extended periods, I have become an expert at noticing subtle changes in mood, alertness, vision, and other senses. My personal experience helps me understand how a supplement works, and gives me additional insights into its potential clinical role. This, combined with interviews with patients and doctors, and results from clinical studies, provides me with a more comprehensive understanding than relying exclusively on research findings.

I do wish to mention that my personal experience is obviously quite subjective, and your response could be different. Many factors could influence a person's experience, including dosage, timing, existing medical conditions, age, sex, and interactions with other nutrients and medicines. Not all brands are the same, either. There could be different amounts of ingredients in different products sold over the counter, due to the particular method of laboratory synthesis and the source of the material or plant.

A WORD ABOUT THE BOOK'S OUTLINE

In Part II of this book you will find a straightforward explanation of how brain cells work and the function of several brain chemicals. Part III provides practical suggestions on how to improve one's mind through diet, exercise, and other lifestyle factors. Part IV gives a detailed explanation of how each supplement works and the research supporting its benefits. Once you take a supplement and notice positive results, you may be interested in learning more about it. Part V provides guidelines on which nutrients to take for your particular age group. Finally, Part VI discusses natural therapies for depression, Alzheimer's disease and Parkinson's disease. There's even a chapter on how to sharpen vision.

I have divided the different supplements in Part IV into several categories, such as brain fats, phospholipids, vitamins, antioxidants, mind energizers, amino acids, hormones, and herbs. Please note that there's an overlap in functions between some of the groups. For instance, CoQ10 is listed under "mind energizers," but it can also act as an antioxidant. Many of the B vitamins are involved in dozens of important chemical reactions in the brain and body. Some of the herbs, like ginkgo, can certainly act both as brain energizers and antioxidants.

But before you jump right into finding out what supplements are recommended for your particular age group, I suggest you learn the top ten important principles of a mind-boosting program.

TWO

The Top Ten Mind-Boosting Principles

With the availability of dozens of mind-enhancing supplements, it is tempting for consumers to rush out and buy a variety of them for a self-prescribed regimen. However, this type of trial is best done cautiously. You should be in touch with your health-care provider to make sure these supplements will not interfere with any of your existing medical conditions or interact with prescription medicines.

There are ten important concepts that I propose in this book regarding supplementation with natural nutrients. It's very important that you review these concepts before you start your mind-boosting program.

1. An Engine Alone Does Not Run a Car.

"If you had to take only one pill, which one would be your choice?" This is a question I am frequently asked. I often reply that a multivitamin and -mineral complex would be my first choice, but, due to the complexities of the human brain, it is too simple to think that one supplement or drug is the complete answer to improving brain function or treating a psychiatric illness. This would be tantamount to asserting that an engine is all that is necessary to run a car. As we all know, a car needs tires, a steering wheel, a carburetor, oil, and hundreds of parts to work at all, let alone work efficiently. A car could have the best engine in the world, but if one of the tires is flat, it's not going to travel too far. Likewise, the approach to improving brain function does not rest on supplying one nutrient in a large dose, but rather depends on our ability to combine positive lifestyle habits with the proper mix of nutrients, and in their right dosages.

Your brain needs a variety of nutrients in small dosages rather than one nutrient in a high dose. In Western medicine, doctors often prescribe one or two medicines in the treatment of medical and psychiatric conditions, whereas in Eastern medicine—Chinese and Indian—most of their formulations include a combination of small amounts of different herbs and nutrients. Eastern doctors learned centuries ago that some medical conditions respond better to the combination of several substances, rather than to just one. Providing a high dose of one nutrient alone may upset the balance of the complex biochemical interactions of the brain. Doctors and patients are often looking for the magic pill that, alone, will cure all ills. The human body is too complicated, with too many biochemical reactions occurring every instant, for one pill to be the answer to all problems. The answer lies in intelligently combining a variety of solutions.

2. Sometimes Less Is More.

Each nutrient has its ideal dosage. If you take more than your brain needs, this could actually lead to a negative reaction. You may not think as clearly, or you may feel distracted, restless, overstimulated, anxious, and irritable. Caution is also advised when combining two or more nutrients since their effects may be cumulative. Hence, when you add a second nutrient, you may need to reduce the dosage of the first one. Keep in mind that caffeine (in coffee, tea, sodas, or chocolate) can have an cumulative effect when combined with nutrients that are stimulants. This could lead to excessive alertness, irritability, or anxiety.

3. Start Low.

You can't always predict how your brain and body will react to a supplement. Start with a small dose and gradually increase it over the next few days. Keep in mind that many researchers doing studies with brain boosters give a high dose in order to elicit a measurable response. These studies are often brief. If you plan to take these nutrients for prolonged periods, your need may be a fraction of the dosage used by the researchers. There is a very wide range of individual response to nutrients.

By starting low and gradually increasing the dosage, potential side effects can be avoided or minimized. You will find that some of the dosages for nutrients listed in this book are much lower than those recommended in some health publications or by some doctors. Since the basic premise of this book is that we all need a variety of different nutrients in order for our brain to function optimally, the required dosage of each should remain low in order to avoid untoward interactions. This is true in regard to the combination of antioxidants because many of them help protect each other from being destroyed; therefore less of each is needed when many are combined. Excessively high dosages of antioxidants can be counterproductive and can lead to what's called pro-oxidation. Dosages also need to be kept low when combining stimulants since their effects are additive. Too many stimulants can cause irritability, insomnia, elevated body temperature, and even heart palpitations.

Over my many years of practicing medicine, I have become much more cautious about dosages. As physicians and individuals, we often blindly follow the recommendations on the package provided by drug or vitamin companies, not appreciating the fact that each person is unique. Some people are very sensitive to even a minute dose of a medicine or nutrient. In some cases the dosage present in the pills you purchase may be excessive and you will need to break a pill in small pieces or open a capsule and take a small portion. For instance, in Chapter 14 I recommend the use of 1 to 5 mg of pregnenolone as replacement therapy, even though some pregnenolone pills sold in vitamin stores come in 50 mg doses.

4. Tolerance Is Possible.

Your brain can build a tolerance to some nutrients if they are used regularly. For instance, I have observed clinically that melatonin does not work well as a sleep aid if used every night. Perhaps there's a reduction in the number of receptors on brain cells for melatonin if they are exposed to high dosages on a regular basis. Hence you will often come across a recommendation that you use a particular nutrient only once or twice a week. Occasionally, take a break ("nutrient, herb, or hormone holiday") from a particular supplement for a few weeks. You may also alternate between similar-functioning supplements on a daily, weekly, or monthly basis. Regular, high-dosage use of a nutrient or hormone could cause feedback inhibition; this means that the body could shut off its own production of the nutrient or hormone if too high of a dose is given on a daily basis for prolonged periods. Note, however, that this is not a common occurrence.

5. Timing Is Crucial.

A supplement can help boost brain power if taken at the right time of day, or it can interfere with brain health if taken at an inappropriate time. Most of the supplements discussed in this book cause alertness and are best taken early in the day. You can either take the whole dose in the morning, or take most of the dose in the morning and the rest midday. If you take a pill that has a stimulant effect in the afternoon or evening, your sleep may be interrupted and you will be worse off for it. Keep in mind that caffeine—in coffee, tea, or chocolate—adds to alertness and stimulation. For obvious reasons, supplements that cause drowsiness, such as melatonin, should be taken at night.

6. Choose the Right Supplement for the Right Setting.

You could have a pleasant or unpleasant experience taking a supplement, depending on your setting. For instance, if you take a high dose of a nutrient that acts as a stimulant and you have to be indoors the whole day at your desk, you may feel restless and irritable. By contrast, if you happen to take this energizer on a weekend and you have the opportunity to walk on a trail by a river, or stroll in a museum, antique store, or gallery, you may have a wonderful time appreciating the beauty while feeling full of vigor. The importance of setting and timing also applies to some of the herbs. For instance, Asian ginseng increases body temperature and is best suited for cold days, while American ginseng has more of a cooling effect and is best suited for warm days. Therefore, it's not only important that you choose the right supplement, or combination of nutrients, but also that you choose the right circumstance, day, time, and setting.

Some of the nutrients discussed in this book that act as stimulants include tyrosine, phenylalanine, St. John's wort, DHEA, pregnenolone, androstenedione, choline, ginseng, ginkgo, coenzyme Q10, SAMe, TMG, DMG, ALC, DMAE, lipoic acid, and high doses of B vitamins. When combined, their effects can be cumulative and lead to overstimulation or insomnia.

7. Some Nutrients Can Accumulate in the Brain and Body.

Some supplements can, over time, accumulate in brain cells, organs, and tissues. This means that with time you may need less of these supplements, not more. Evaluate your supplements regularly and reduce the dosages if you find that you are becoming overstimulated or are having side effects.

8. Brain Supplements Influence the Whole Body.

When you take the nutrients discussed in this book for cognitive enhancement purposes, they will not only have an effect on the brain, but on numerous bodily organs and tissues. Most of the nutrients and herbs I have included in this book have positive effects on physical and mental health. However, high dosages of some, when used carelessly and indiscriminately, could have undesirable physical effects. You can find detailed information on particular nutrient side effects in Part IV.

9. Some Natural Supplements Have Not Been Thoroughly Tested.

In 1994, the Congress of the United States passed a dietary-supplement law that allowed the entry of new supplements to the market without needing approval from the FDA. Ever since the easing of dietary-supplement laws, the health industry has had virtual carte blanche to introduce a wide variety of nutrients and herbal extracts. Many vitamin companies are in a quandary when a new supplement becomes available. Should they wait until more studies are published on the product's safety, or should they introduce the product right away? If they wait too long, other companies could begin to distribute the product and gain a large market share. Therefore, in the mad rush to market products as soon as possible in order to beat the competition, many supplements become available to the public when little is known about their long-term effects. Do not assume that just because a nutrient bottle is within easy reach on a store shelf that many studies have been done to support its efficacy or safety. Some of these supplements have powerful, drug-like effects—both positive and negative.

10. Train Your Neurons.

You could take the most powerful mind boosters ever invented, but if you don't engage in mental activities such as reading, learning, thinking, and creating, you will get only a fraction of the potential benefits from these supplements. Part III will provide you with some practical tips on how to exercise your brain, along with a discussion of a few lifestyle habits regarding diet, positive mental attitude, deep sleep, and stress reduction. Supplements can have dramatic benefits, but are only the icing on the cake (except in older individuals who are often deficient in nutrients, or in the treatment of a medical or neurological disorder). Even though I'm very excited about the benefits of the nutrients discussed in this book, I still feel that the most important steps you can take for optimal brain health are to cultivate positive lifestyle habits, get regular sleep, and engage in continuous mental stimulation.

PART II

Your Brain—An Owner's Guide

THREE

The ABCs of the Brain

If you're reading this book, it's apparent that you have a significant interest in finding natural ways to improve your mental performance or to treat a particular neurological condition. In order to achieve these goals more reliably, it helps to have a basic knowledge of the structure of the brain and how this incredibly complex organ works. The chapter explains the function of brain cells and discusses changes that occur in these cells during normal aging. The more we learn about how the brain works, the better we can improve its potential.

THE NEURON

Everything in our bodies—muscles, organs, skin, and bones—is made of tiny cells. This is also true of the brain. The cells in the brain are called **neurons**. An average brain has about one hundred billion neurons (fifteen times the population of the world). In addition to neurons, about nine hundred billion **glial cells** are present in the brain. These glial cells surround and nutritionally support neurons.

COMMON TERMS USED IN THIS CHAPTER

CELL—the smallest organized unit of living structure in the body.

CELL MEMBRANE—a thin layer, consisting mostly of phospholipids, that surrounds and encloses each cell.

CENTRAL NERVOUS SYSTEM—the brain, along with the nerves of the spinal cord. The *peripheral nervous system* refers to the nerves outside of the central nervous system, such as the nerves in the arms and legs.

CEREBRUM—the top, main part of the brain, consisting of left and right sides. It controls voluntary thoughts and movements.

CEREBRAL CORTEX—the outer part of the cerebrum, the main thinking area of the brain.

COGNITION—mental activities such as thinking, memory, perception, judgment, and learning.

DENDRITE—the treelike branching arms of a neuron.

NEURON—a cell in the brain. There are billions of neurons in the brain that communicate with each other with neurotransmitters through connections called **synapses**.

NEUROTRANSMITTER—a biochemical substance, such as serotonin, dopamine, or acetylcholine, that relays messages from one neuron to another.

PHOSPHOLIPIDS—fatty acids combined with the mineral phosphorus and other compounds. Phospholipids are the primary constituents of a cell membrane.

SYNAPSE—the point of contact between two neurons, where nerve impulses are transmitted from one to the other.

Neuron-to-Neuron Communication

Neurons communicate with each other through electrical impulses and chemicals. These chemicals are called **neurotransmitters**. A typical neuron has thousands of connections, called **synapses**, with neighboring neurons.

Every single external stimulation that enters through our five senses

Figure 3.1—Neuron-to-Neuron Communication

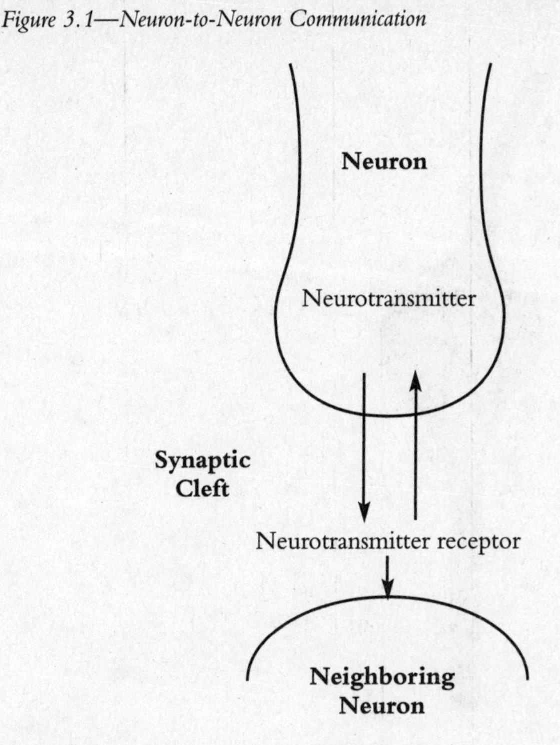

Brain cells communicate with each other through thousands of connections at sites called synapses.

(sight, hearing, smell, touch, and taste) causes tiny electrical nerve impulses and the release of minute amounts of neurotransmitters. At present, about a hundred or so different neurotransmitters have been identified. Some of these include serotonin, dopamine, norepinephrine, and acetylcholine.

Neurotransmitters, such as serotonin, produce their effects by interacting with appropriate receptors located on "next-door neighbor" neurons (see Figures 3.1 and 3.2). As is the case with some of the neurotransmitters, serotonin is made in brain cells and stored in small

Figure 3.2—Synaptic Cleft

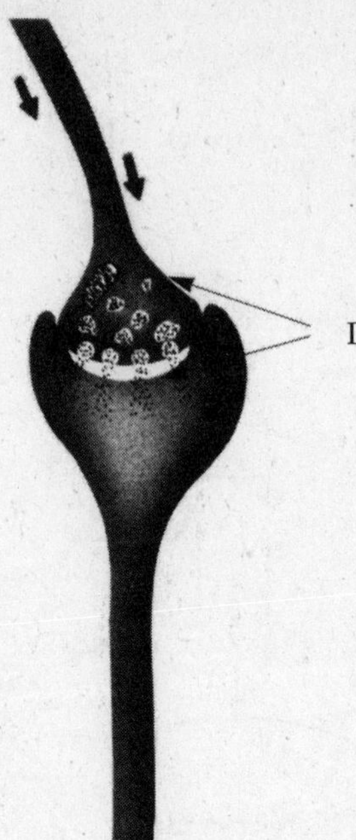

A single nerve may make up to 20,000 connections with other cells. The place where these cells connect is called the synapse. The portion of the nerve making the connection is called the synaptic membrane. This part of the nerve has a higher concentration of the brain-fat DHA than almost any tissue in the body.

enclosures within the cells called **vesicles**. When a neuron is stimulated, the vesicles open at the edge of the neuron, and serotonin is released outside of the neuron into a tiny space near an adjoining neuron. This space is called a **synaptic cleft**. Thereafter, serotonin will interact with various serotonin receptors located on these adjoining brain cells and influence their function.

After serotonin is released into the synaptic cleft, it can either be taken back into the neuron that released it in the first place (a process called "reuptake"), or it can be broken down by enzymes located within the synaptic cleft. In general, the most common way that ends serotonin action in the synaptic cleft is its reuptake. Selective serotonin reuptake inhibitors (SSRIs), such as Prozac, increase the amount of serotonin in the synaptic cleft by preventing this reuptake.

COMPOSITION OF THE CELL MEMBRANE

It has been well established that changing levels of neurotransmitters in the brain influence mood, memory, and mental function; not as clearly recognized is the fact that altering the composition of brain-cell membranes can also influence many aspects of brain function. A discussion of cell membranes is important because many of the nutrients discussed in this book, such as fish oils and phospholipids, have an effect by altering the **cell membrane** of brain cells.

Each neuron is enclosed within a cell membrane, which separates the inside of the cell from the outside (see Figure 3.3). The cell membrane serves as a barrier, allowing certain necessary compounds to come in, while restricting the entry of undesirable substances. Receptors for many brain chemicals are also found on the membrane. The composition of this membrane consists mostly of different types of lipids (or fats), which include phosphatidylcholine (PC), phosphatidylserine (PS), and other lipids. Therefore, as you can guess, manipulation of the composition of the lipids of cell membranes can influence the function of neurons. The composition of a cell membrane is in a constant state of flux, influenced by diet, stress, and the immune system.

The cell membrane has two layers, an inner one facing the inside of the cell, and an outer one facing the outside. The composition of the membrane includes several types of compounds. The two most common groups include phospholipids and sterols (Aloia 1988). Phospholipids are lipids made up mostly by fatty acids, amino acids, and the mineral phosphorus. The major types of phospholipids include phosphatidylcholine (PC, or lecithin), comprising about 30 percent

Figure 3.3—Cell Membrane

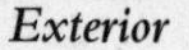

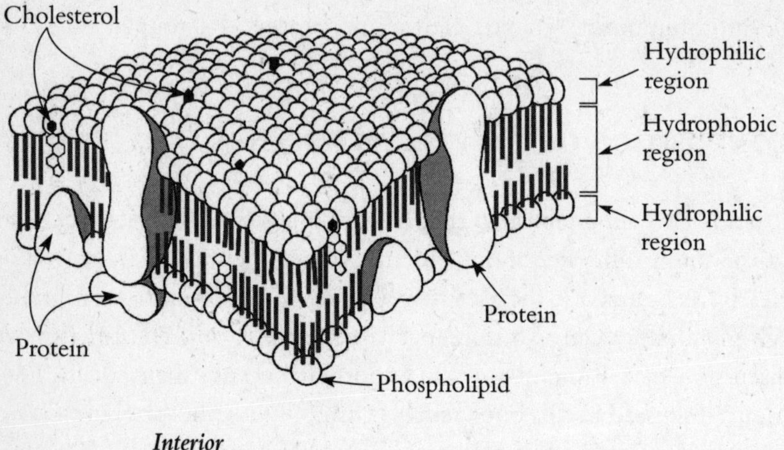

The lining of a cell membrane is composed mostly of fatty acids. The types of fatty acids present are partially influenced by diet.

of the lipid content of the brain; phosphatidylethanolamine (PE), comprising about 27 percent of the lipid content of the brain; and phosphatidylserine (PS), comprising less than 10 percent of the lipid content of the brain (Suzuki 1981). Sterols include cholesterol, comprising about 20 percent of the lipid content of the brain. Cholesterol forms an important part of brain structure and is the precursor from which the steroid hormones, such as DHEA, progesterone, estrogen, and testosterone, are formed.

As you can see in Figure 3.4, the composition of the cell membrane influences the structure of neurotransmitter receptors. Figure 3.5 provides an overall perspective, from the brain down to the neuron, the cell membrane, phospholipids, and fatty acids.

Figure 3.4—Receptor on Cell Membrane

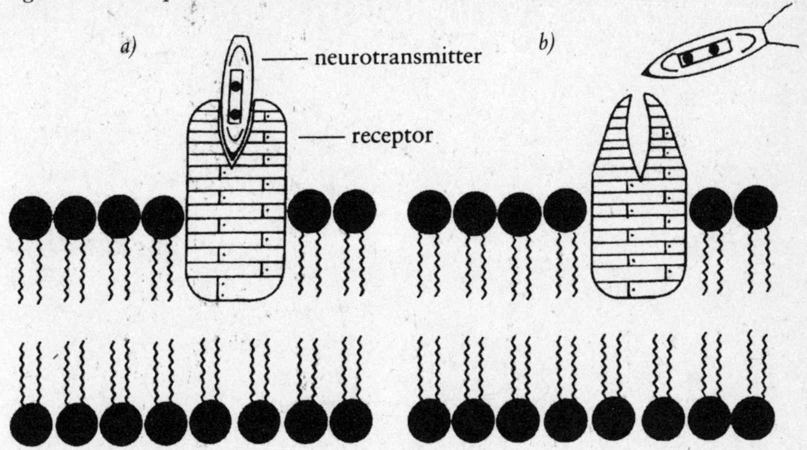

Nerve cells communicate by releasing neurotransmitters into the synaptic space. While in this space, the neurotransmitter molecules seek a "port," or receptor, into which they neatly fit. The ability to "dock" depends upon the shape of both the neurotransmitter and the receptor. Fatty-acid balance affects the shape of the dock (receptor), which may make it difficult for the neurotransmitter (ship) to fit. This may slow nerve communication and affect many aspects of brain function. Part *a)* shows the proper "fit" of the ship in the dock. Part *b)* illustrates how changing the dock's shape prevents the ship from docking.

TRAINING NEURONS

Every single thought or emotion you experience is associated with tiny electrical nerve impulses and the release of minute amounts of neurotransmitters between neurons. Reading this sentence is causing electrical nerve impulses and the release of neurotransmitters in certain parts of your brain. Your eyes are sensing the shapes of the letters, and the information is then relayed to your cerebral cortex. These letters and words are interpreted in the brain, and then converted into thoughts. These thoughts are in turn stored as memory. The nature of your thoughts is dependent on your genetic makeup, prior learn-

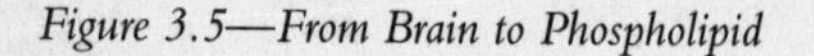

Figure 3.5—From Brain to Phospholipid

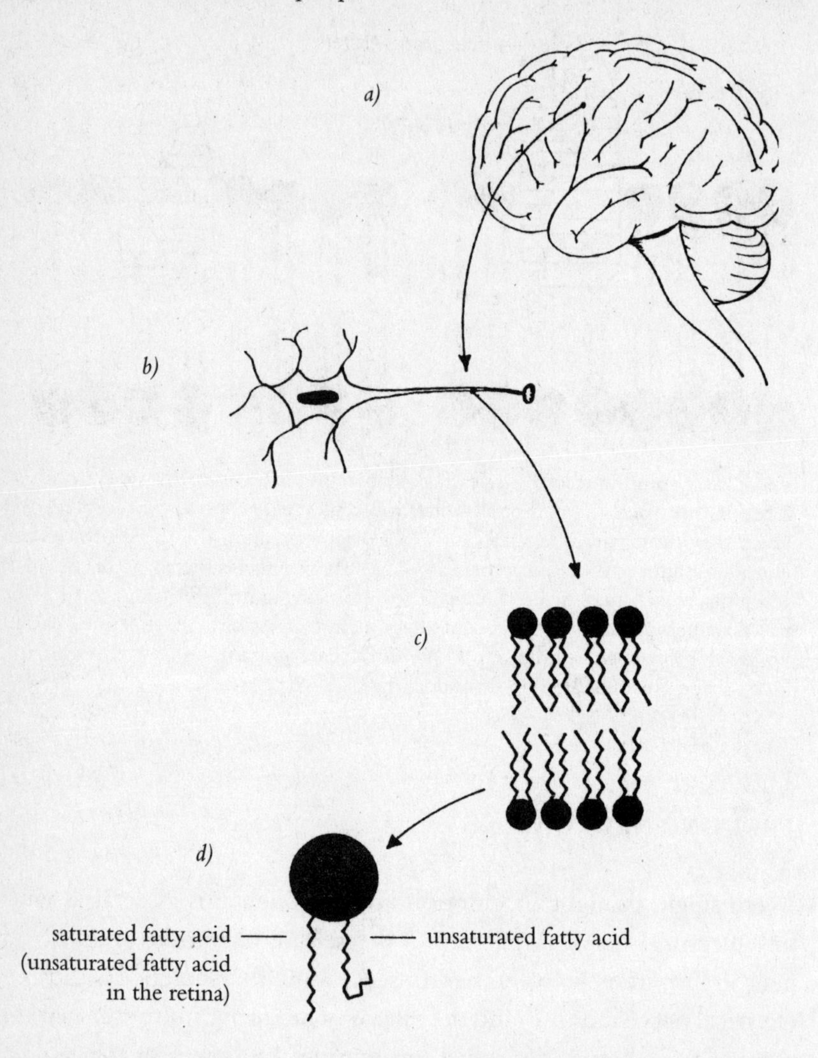

The brain is reduced here into simpler and simpler components eventually revealing the location of the fatty acids. This system is highly organized: *a)* the brain; *b)* the nerve cell with a cutaway of the cell membrane, or covering; *c)* the membrane's two layers, in which the fatty acid "tails" face the interior of the membrane; *d)* a single phospholipid molecule containing one saturated fat (straight) and one unsaturated fatty acid (curved). In the brain, the unsaturated fatty acid is usually DHA or AA. In the retina, both positions typically contain the unsaturated fatty acid DHA.

ing, experience, and memory. Everyone has a different brain and no two individuals reading this paragraph will have the same exact thoughts. Memory is mostly due to the strengthening of connections between neurons, and the formation of protein molecules within neurons. A newly formed memory often involves interactions between hundreds and thousands of neurons. If this new encoding doesn't get used, it will soon fade. But if you continue to reactivate the information that you have stored—for instance, by rereading this sentence—the connections become reinforced. There are microscopic anatomical (physical) changes going on in your brain at this moment as a result of your reading this paragraph.

Many parts of the brain are involved in the process of memory acquisition and storage, particularly the **cerebral cortex** (which is the outer part of the brain) and the **hippocampus** (a structure located deep in the brain). The hippocampus is involved mostly in short-term memory processing and is often one of the first areas damaged in Alzheimer's disease.

A fascinating experiment studied two groups of mice (Gispen 1993). The first group was placed in a cage and had no mental stimulation; they chaise-lounged all day. The second group was trained to run through mazes. After a few weeks, the neurons of the trained mice were compared to those of the untrained group with an electron microscope. There was a noticeable difference. The group that had been trained had wider and longer **dendrites** (the treelike communicating arms between neurons) and more synapses. Later, the trained group was taken out of the stimulating environment and placed in cages without stimulation. At the end of a few weeks, their brains were examined. The dendrites and synapses appeared similar to the group that had not been trained. Their neurons had shrunk back to their original size.

Other studies have confirmed that when toys are placed in cages of laboratory animals, dendrites branch out and synaptic connections increase in as little as four days (Black 1991). The brain is living tissue, similar to a muscle, in that it grows and becomes more efficient the more it is used. The brain grows and changes depending on its stimulation. It can become smarter, improve its capacity for memory and creativity, and generally improve in any direction in which it is stimulated. A mind can be channeled in any of several directions, talents, or occupations. Anyone can become smarter and more creative with effort. Fortunately, we can help our brains perform better with the intelligent use of nutritional supplements, especially as we get older.

What Happens When the Brain Gets Old?

A number of changes occur in the brain as we age. The most obvious include

- Deterioration and loss of brain cells, dendrites, synapses, and receptors
- Deterioration of cell membranes
- A decline or alterations in hormone levels
- A decline or alterations in levels of brain chemicals
- Malfunction of the energy-production system in cells
- A decrease in blood flow to the brain and within the brain, often as a consequence of atherosclerosis (hardening of the arteries), or small and large strokes
- Accumulation of waste products such as lipofuscin within brain cells

What Can You Do to Keep Your Mind Young?

In order to restore mental performance, many of these age-related changes need to be slowed and even reversed. Fortunately, this is possible. Part III of this book gives practical advice on how to train your mind in order to maintain healthy neurons, dendrites, and synapses. Many of the mind boosters that have been introduced in the past few years are able to help the brain stay young and sharp. For instance, cell membranes may be restored by the fatty acids and phospholipids discussed in Chapters 7 and 8, respectively. Accumulation of waste products can be reduced by the antioxidants mentioned in

Chapter 11. The energy-production system can be improved by providing some of the mind energizers discussed in Chapter 12. Hormone levels can be restored, as reviewed in Chapter 14. Ginkgo and vinpocetine, two herbal extracts discussed in Chapter 15, can improve blood flow to the brain. As you can see, there are many steps we can take to keep our mind as young as possible.

FOUR

Brain Chemistry Made Simple

The information you gather when you look, hear, taste, touch, and smell, is processed in your brain through electrical and chemical messengers. The chemical messengers that help brain cells communicate with each other are called **neurotransmitters**. Dozens of substances or chemicals in the brain—amines, amino acids, minerals, hormones, and peptides—act as neurotransmitters, influencing memory, mood, alertness, and thinking. A review of all of these neurotransmitters is not necessary for the purposes of this book. However, a brief explanation of some of the important neurotransmitters will make it easier for you to understand how the natural supplements discussed in this book affect the mind. It will also help you choose the right supplements for your particular needs.

Unless you are already familiar with some of these neurotransmitters, you may find the information in this chapter to be very detailed. In that case, I recommend you use this chapter as a reference. Whenever you take a nutrient that you find helpful, your interest in learning more about its chemistry and function will motivate you to return to this chapter and delve into its biochemistry in more detail.

A BRIEF SUMMARY OF BRAIN CHEMICALS AND THEIR MAJOR FUNCTIONS

- Acetylcholine helps with memory and learning.
- Dopamine is primarily responsible for sex drive, mood, alertness, and movement.
- Norepinephrine and epinephrine influence alertness, arousal, and mood.
- Serotonin is involved in mood, appetite control, emotional balance, and impulse control.
- GABA helps with relaxation and sedation.

Please keep in mind that these are simplifications. The functions of these neurotransmitters often overlap and they may have different effects in different parts of the brain.

ACETYLCHOLINE

Acetylcholine was the very first neurotransmitter to be identified, back in the early 1900s. It is made simply from choline and a two-carbon molecule called acetyl. Acetylcholine plays numerous roles in the nervous system. In the brain, acetylcholine is involved in learning and memory. Chapter 8 discusses how supplements such as choline and CDP-choline influence levels of acetylcholine.

Once produced, acetylcholine is stored in brain cells and released into the synaptic cleft upon stimulation. When released into the synaptic cleft, the enzyme acetylcholinesterase breaks acetylcholine back down into choline and acetyl. In Alzheimer's disease, there is a shortage of acetylcholine, and one of the ways doctors have tried to increase the levels of this neurotransmitter is by prescribing drugs, such as tacrine, that inhibit the enzyme acetylcholinesterase. In Chapter 15

I discuss an alternative to these drugs, a Chinese herbal extract called huperzine A, that also inhibits this enzyme.

DOPAMINE

A number of psychiatric disorders, particularly schizophrenia, Parkinson's disease, and mood disorders, are attributed to imbalances in dopamine levels. Elevation of dopamine levels often leads to an improvement in mood, alertness, and sex drive, and perhaps even an enhancement in verbal fluency and creativity. Dopamine is made from the amino acid tyrosine (see Figure 4.1). Once produced, dopamine can in turn convert into the brain chemicals norepinephrine and epinephrine.

When released into the synaptic cleft, dopamine is broken down by the enzyme monoamine oxidase (MAO). This is an important point to keep in mind since many pharmaceutical drugs take advantage of this reaction. In fact, there are drugs that block the activity of MAO, and hence are known as "MAO inhibitors." There are two types of MAO inhibitors—type A and type B. They can both act as antidepressants, and the type-B inhibitors are also used to treat Parkinson's disease. Selegiline (or deprenyl) is a well-known pharmaceutical MAO type-B inhibitor. Ingestion of selegiline leads to arousal, alertness, and an increase in sexual drive.

A decline in dopamine activity in the brain is linked to cognitive (learning and memory) and movement problems in those with Parkinson's disease. In upcoming chapters, I will discuss how the amino acids phenylalanine and tyrosine, along with the nutrient nicotinamide adenosine dinucleotide (NADH) and some of the B vitamins, influence the production of dopamine.

Figure 4.1—The Making of Dopamine and Norepinephrine from Amino Acids

Phenylalanine

▼ Nicotinamide adenosine dinucleotide (NADH)

Tyrosine

▼ Vitamin C

L-Dopa

▼ Vitamin B_6

Dopamine

▼ Vitamin C

Norepinephrine

▼ methyl donors

Epinephrine

NOREPINEPHRINE AND EPINEPHRINE

As you can see in Figure 4.1, the amino acids phenylalanine and tyrosine are converted into dopamine. Dopamine, in turn, is converted into norepinephrine and then epinephrine. As can be predicted from this figure, the ingestion of tyrosine elevates dopamine and norepinephrine levels, and hence will lead to alertness and mood elevation. Excess amounts of these neurotransmitters raise blood pressure, increase heart rate, and cause anxiety, irritability, and insomnia. Certain pharmaceutical antidepressants elevate mood and enhance arousal by increasing levels of norepinephrine and epinephrine.

Both phenylalanine and tyrosine are available over-the-counter, and they are discussed in Chapter 13. Several enzymes are required to make the conversion from phenylalanine to epinephrine, and these enzymes require helpers, such as vitamins and nutrients. Figure 4.1 shows several of these nutrients. For instance, vitamin B_6 helps convert L-dopa to dopamine, while vitamin C helps convert dopamine to norepinephrine.

SEROTONIN

Serotonin is the most widely studied neurotransmitter since it helps regulate a vast range of psychological and biological functions. Serotonin (5-hydroxytryptamine or 5-HT) was first identified in 1948. The wide extent of psychological functions regulated by serotonin involves mood, anxiety, arousal, aggression, and thinking abilities. You may recall that other brain chemicals, such as dopamine and norepinephrine, also influence mood and arousal. However, serotonin generally has different effects. For instance, excess amounts of serotonin cause relaxation, sedation, and a decrease in sexual drive.

Prozac, a common antidepressant, elevates serotonin levels, and perhaps influences the levels of other brain chemicals. There is an over-the-counter nutrient called 5-hydroxytryptophan (5-HTP) that is the immediate precursor to serotonin and can, in some cases, temporarily substitute for serotonin-influencing drugs (see Chapter 13). Some research suggests that perhaps the herbal antidepressant St. John's wort also works by elevating levels of serotonin in the brain.

Disruption of the normal functioning of the serotonergic system leads to a number of psychiatric conditions, which include anxiety disorders, depression, improper social behavior, and sexual aberrations. Common medical conditions associated with disruption of the serotonergic system include disturbance in the sleep-wake cycle, obesity or eating disorders, and chronic pain.

Figure 4.2 shows that the starting point in the production of serotonin is tryptophan, one of the amino acids we ingest through food, particularly meat, fish, and other protein foods. If not enough tryptophan is supplied to the brain, serotonin levels drop. Furthermore,

Figure 4.2—The Making of Serotonin

Tryptophan
▼
5-Hydroxytryptophan
▼ **Vitamin B_6**
Serotonin
▼ **methyl donors**
Melatonin

in order for tryptophan to enter the brain, it has to be transported across the blood-brain barrier by a carrier protein. This carrier protein is also used by other amino acids, including phenylalanine and tyrosine, two amino acids that convert in the brain to dopamine and norepinephrine. Imagine this carrier as a small canoe that can carry only one person across a lake at a time. There's always competition between the different amino acids to jump on the canoe. Therefore, brain levels of tryptophan are not only determined by the concentration of tryptophan in the bloodstream, but also by the concentration of competing amino acids.

Once tryptophan enters the brain, it can go into brain cells and be converted into 5-HTP and then into serotonin. After serotonin is made, the pineal gland is able to convert it at night into the sleep hormone melatonin. Other areas of the brain don't have the necessary enzymes to make this conversion.

GABA

Gamma-aminobutyric acid, discovered in 1950, is the most important and widespread inhibitory neurotransmitter in the brain. Excitation in the brain must be balanced with inhibition. Too much excitation can lead to restlessness, irritability, insomnia, and even seizures. GABA is able to induce relaxation, analgesia, and sleep. Barbiturates and benzodiazepines are known to stimulate GABA receptors, and hence induce relaxation. Several neurological disorders, such as epilepsy, sleep disorders, and Parkinson's disease are affected by this neurotransmitter.

GABA is made in the brain from the amino acid glutamate with the aid of vitamin B_6. GABA is available as a supplement in vitamin stores, but taking it in pill form is not an effective way to raise brain levels of this neurotransmitter because GABA cannot easily cross the blood-brain barrier. Companies are searching for ways to place GABA in an oil base in order to ease its entry across this barrier.

ADDITIONAL NEUROTRANSMITTERS

There are dozens of other chemicals—amino acids, peptides, and hormones—found in the brain that influence mood and cognition. These include glutamate, histamine, endorphins, enkephalins, growth hormone, vasopressin, prolactin, oxytocin, nitric oxide, prostaglandins, and others. It's very likely that many of the supplements discussed in this book affect these chemicals, and further research will certainly identify these biochemical processes.

THE CONNECTION BETWEEN THE BRAIN AND THE IMMUNE SYSTEM

As if all of the chemicals discussed above weren't enough, there are many messengers—such as cytokines—that are released by the immune system and influence brain cells and levels of neurotransmitters; some of these cytokines are interleukins, interferons, and tumor necrosis factor. Hence, a healthy immune system is necessary for a well-functioning brain. The brain can, in turn, release chemicals and hormones that influence the immune system. For instance, there are serotonin receptors on white blood cells. The brain-immune connection is a two-way affair. If you've ever had a bad case of the flu and felt fatigued and depressed for a few days afterward, you experienced the immediate negative effects of certain cytokines on your brain cells and neurotransmitters. If you've ever been stressed and come down with a cold, you perhaps realized the immune-suppressing effect of certain brain chemicals and hormones released by the brain as a consequence of stress.

Summary

I find brain chemistry fascinating, particularly since we now have access to a number of natural supplements that can help us manipulate our neurotransmitters. By understanding brain chemistry and how supplements work, we can more effectively improve our mental capacities and performance.

PART III

Lifestyle Habits for a Long-Lasting Brain

FIVE

How to Cultivate a Naturally Healthy Mind

In this book I focus on natural, mind-boosting supplements, but any book that discusses mental health must address the significant influence of diet and lifestyle. We may use the most powerful mind boosters available, but if we don't exercise the brain and body, eat the right foods, continue on a path of emotional growth, cultivate healthy relationships, and have good sleeping patterns, we will not reap the full benefits of the supplements.

We live in a world that places enormous demands on our mental abilities. Continually expanding our mind and memory capacity is crucial to successful adaptation to this ever-changing, informational society. Enhancing our mental capacity helps us advance in our career, leading to more work satisfaction, higher income, greater travel and leisure opportunities, less stress, and more autonomy.

An increase in intelligence and a large fund of knowledge give us an improved sense of self-confidence. As our topics of interest and discussion increase, so can the number and variety of social contacts. Knowledge also improves our ability to foresee future political, economic, and historical trends.

The more we learn, the more we wish to continue learning. Understanding the world is like assembling a jigsaw puzzle. The more pieces we fit, the clearer the image and the greater the urge to learn and fill in even more pieces. Increasing one's knowledge can be compared to an avalanche: once the process starts, it gathers a momentum of its own. Perseverance and some initial prompting are required, but the rewards soon pay off. Minds are kept young by continual use, and mentally active people live longer. I consider mind-enhancement to be a lifelong process. Centuries ago René Descartes said, "It is not enough to have a good mind. The main thing is to use it well." The march of intellect need not halt soon after framing the high school or college diploma.

EMOTIONAL CONNECTIONS

During this process of intellectual enhancement, keep in mind that we also need to grow emotionally. Although supplements can help provide the basic ingredients for proper mental functioning, they cannot, on their own, help us develop healthy relationships. In order for us to feel truly fulfilled, it helps to cultivate healthy connections on multiple levels.

The need for connection may be fulfilled in several ways. On a personal level, we can connect with fellow human beings through friendship, physical intimacy, romance, marriage, and family. We can also satisfy our need for connection with cats, dogs, other animals, and nature as a whole. We satisfy the urge to belong to something larger than ourselves by joining religious, humanistic, philosophic, or any number of community groups. As a rule, the more ways we connect, the happier we become.

Supplements can sometimes help in this regard by lifting our mood and improving our motivation to become social and interact with others.

EXERCISE

If you've reached middle age—or passed it—and have never exercised regularly, it's not too late to start. Maintaining the exercise habit, or taking up light-to-moderate physical activity later in life, helps us live longer. Physical activity improves mental function by inducing the growth of capillaries (tiny blood vessels) in the brain, which helps many nutrients reach neurons. This is important because the aging process leads to a decrease in blood supply to the brain.

Physical exercise also leads to deep sleep. During deep sleep, the brain gets a chance to consolidate memory and rebalance hormones and brain chemicals to get us ready for a new day.

LEARN HOW TO LEARN

Learning is an art that improves with time. There are several practical steps you can take to acquire more knowledge.

The more words we learn, the more aware we become of our surroundings. Look up unfamiliar words in the dictionary. Jot a reminder by the word to indicate where you encountered it, whether in a book, a magazine, a newspaper, or in conversation. For example, if you come across a new word while reading the *New York Times*, write *NYT* by the word in the dictionary. If you come across the word in a book, write the title of the book by the word. Next time you look up the same word, the previous annotation will help you form an association, and you will have an easier time remembering the word. There are many occasions when I look up a word in my dictionary and realize I have noted it before. I make a special effort to remember this word in order to learn it once and for all. The odds are high that I will encounter this word again in the future. Almost every page of my *Webster's Dictionary* has some notation on it. Another great way to stimulate the mind and learn new words is to do crossword puzzles.

Once we start learning new words, it is a pleasant surprise when we encounter the same words again because each new word reinforces a memory. Consider the dictionary or encyclopedia one of your most interesting friends. "Words form the thread on which we string our experiences," summarized Aldous Huxley, the British philosopher.

If you have time, read a brief history of the world, and improve your geographical knowledge—buy an atlas and look up the major countries and their capitals. Whenever you encounter the name of a city you have not heard before, look for it in an atlas. A review of the important figures in literature, art, and music will be very helpful. *Jeopardy!* is a good television show to watch. This game is a great mental exercise for improving memory and recall, and you can learn an incredible amount of information that you will likely come across again in your daily life. I often program my VCR to tape the show, and when I have time, I sit down to review the episodes. If I can't think of the answer, I put the tape on pause for a few seconds to think hard and to try to remember. Watching *Jeopardy!* or playing games involving trivia or recall can significantly enhance your memory and intelligence. Mind-boosting supplements make a great synergistic combination with games that stimulate thinking and recall.

You may also find that your ability to be funny improves as you learn more words and increase your mental capacity. Your mind will start thinking faster. Making a joke or saying something witty becomes easier, since words, ideas, and trivial details are easily accessible.

CULTIVATE YOUR CREATIVITY

"The barriers are not erected," wrote Ludwig van Beethoven, "which shall say to aspiring talent, 'thus far and no farther.' "

Creativity, an expression of one's individuality, demands self-discipline—that is, motivation, effort, and perseverance. You don't know where your talents will lead if you don't make the initial effort to start. Writing and English were two of my weakest subjects in high school and college; I always excelled in mathematics and science. The last thing on my mind in medical school and residency was to be a medical writer. I would never have guessed when I published my first book that I had the potential to be a prolific writer.

There is a strong drive in humans to create, construct, or invent. The end product might be a piece of art, a musical score, a poem, a house, or simply a better-tasting salad dressing. We can find original ways to approach daily problems. An office worker can write a better memo; a gardener can sculpt new shapes of bushes; a laboratory worker can find a new solution to a project; and a homemaker can find creative ways to shop and balance the family budget. There are countless opportunities in our daily life to be creative.

SAMPLE! EXPLORE! EXPAND!

As we age, there is a tendency to gradually shun novelty and surround ourselves with the familiar. This can lead to getting stuck in a rut.

Planet Earth provides a bounty of sensual and pleasurable potentials, yet we nibble from the edges. We cloister ourselves from new experiences. Our senses are repeatedly reexposed to the same stimuli. We lose touch with our novelty-seeking drive and slope imperceptibly toward the ordinary, the routine, and the unconscious. We wonder why we're not obtaining pleasure and satisfaction from things we used to enjoy. Familiarity turns into routine. One week becomes no different from the week before, or the week after. Eventually, familiarity metamorphoses into a master demanding the same television shows, the same meals, the same vacation spots, the same everything. The pendulum arcs to and fro, seasons come and go, and we continue our downward slump into a rut.

It can happen to any of us. Familiarity, in very subtle ways, numbs our senses and saps our initiative. But there is a way out of this rut. Once we are aware of this trend, we can take steps to turn the tide. A little effort expands our comfort zone. Having made this effort, we realize how easy it is to continue expanding. The first step is the hardest.

In order to keep your mind at its best, add variety to your life. Make the effort to meet new people, engage in good conversation, attend concerts, and take adult classes in art, literature, poetry, music, or painting. What about an acting, dance, or improvisation class? Engage in a new sport. Travel to destinations you don't normally visit. Have you visited all the museums in or near your town or city? Taking handfuls of brain-boosting supplements while reclining on a sofa in front of the tube is not the answer.

But if you are stuck in a rut, some of the nutrients discussed in this book can motivate you to break out of this trend of mental decline and boredom. By improving mood, increasing energy levels, enhancing visual perception, and increasing motivation, these supplements can be the catalysts that get you back to enjoying the beautiful world we live in. While in the process of expanding, we need to remind ourselves to reappreciate and love the familiar, being grateful for everything we already have and are able to do.

SMART EATING

Mental health is, in many ways, linked to physical health. The cardiovascular system supplies blood and oxygen to the brain. When the arteries to the brain are clogged, the blood supply to important neural centers decreases. Cardiovascular disease can often foretell cognitive decline—those who have poor blood flow suffer mental decline faster than those with good vascular health.

Just about every step you take to improve your physical well-being will influence your brain health—especially the right diet. Since the topic of healthy eating has been covered thoroughly in many books and articles, I just wish to make a few important points.

Breakfast is essential for good thinking. Mom was right, after all, when she urged you to eat before going off to school. Dr. David Benton and colleagues from the University of Wales-Swansea, in the United Kingdom, studied the effects of skipping breakfast versus eating breakfast (Benton 1998). Morning fasting was found to adversely affect the ability to recall a word list and stories read aloud, as well as to recall items while counting backward. However, the failure to eat breakfast did not affect performance on an intelligence test. The researchers conclude that breakfast influences tasks requiring aspects of memory, partly through increasing blood-sugar levels. Even a small breakfast snack is enough.

For optimum alertness and brain function, I recommend eating small, frequent meals throughout the day that include a balanced amount of protein, fat, and carbohydrates. Protein helps us stay alert. If you have trouble falling asleep, toward evening you can switch to having more carbohydrates, which help to induce slumber. Good choices of carbohydrates include unprocessed grains, barley, lentils, legumes, vegetables, and fruits. A small amount of pasta is another option.

Here are some other suggestions for a smart diet:

- Reduce your intake of sugar and simple carbohydrates. Most people don't realize that sugars can convert into fats, particularly saturated fatty acids such as palmitic acid. When appropriate, use the natural, no-calorie sweetener stevia as a substitute for sugar.
- Reduce your intake of saturated fats if your diet includes a large amount. However, don't go to an extreme by trying to cut out all saturated fats. Moderation is the key.
- Decrease your intake of fried foods, margarine, and baked goods. These foods contain trans-fatty acids and hydrogenated oils that interfere with the function of good fats.
- Use more olive, canola, and flaxseed oils and less safflower, sunflower, and corn oils. Include more omega-3 fatty acids in the diet, particularly through consumption of fish. If you don't like fish, or don't eat enough marine products, take fish-oil supplements. When purchasing canned tuna or sardines, avoid the ones soaked in soybean oil or other omega-6 oils. For instance, you can eat sardines packed in mustard or tomato sauce, or olive oil.

- Vary your fruit and vegetable intake by purchasing produce that you don't normally eat. Each fruit or vegetable has a unique set of carotenoids and flavonoids. Attempt, on a regular basis, to consume citrus fruits, berries, apricots, grapes, and other fruits. Your vegetable intake should include garlic, onions, green leafy vegetables, yellow- or orange-colored vegetables, tomatoes, and beets.
- Drink a variety of herbal teas instead of just regular tea or coffee. Each morning, have a different type of tea, such as ginger, bilberry, green tea, licorice, peppermint, lemon grass, and so on.
- Drink one or two large glasses of water when you wake up in the morning to help empty the colon.

Dietary choices are ours to make, but unfortunately, we are also influenced by the food choices of our family, friends, and community. For instance, the types of meals served at local restaurants certainly influence our choices. Many of the dishes may be deep-fried. In some areas of the country, fish is very expensive or rarely part of the menu. People who live in small towns or rural areas may be limited in their access to a variety of fruits and vegetables.

A NOTE TO VEGETARIANS

I have many patients who are vegetarians. Some are able to function very well and are able to ingest the right nutrients for optimal health. Others suffer from fatigue and low mood since they may be missing certain nutrients found exclusively in eggs, milk, meat, and fish.

If you're a vegetarian, you may not be getting enough CoQ10, creatine, carnitine, and omega-3 oils. Supplement your diet with flaxseed oil for omega-3s, and take about 10 mg of CoQ10; 100 to 250 mg of carnitine, and about 1 g of creatine on a daily basis. Make sure your intake of protein is adequate. Many vegetarians have a tendency to overconsume carbohydrates at the expense of protein.

THE DEEP SLEEP

Nothing seems to improve memory, mood, and overall cognition like a good night's sleep. If you need help sleeping, once in a while you can use a sleep-inducing supplement such as 5-HTP or melatonin, or the herbs valerian and hops. Here are eight suggestions for a good night's rest:

1. Expose yourself to morning light for at least ten to twenty minutes. Morning light exposure shortens the sleep cycle so that when you go to bed at night it will be easier to fall asleep.
2. Exercise will definitely give you a deeper sleep. The best times to work out are in the late afternoon or early evening. Exercise may delay sleep if performed within three or so hours before bedtime due to arousal and increase in body heat. If you take some of the stimulants discussed in this book, you will definitely need to do some physical activity in order to use up the excess energy, otherwise you will still be stimulated at bedtime, and your sleep will be shallow.
3. Caffeine in any form (sodas, chocolate, coffee, or certain teas, including green tea) is best avoided after dinner. Some individuals may be so sensitive to caffeine's stimulant effects that even drinking coffee at lunch can interfere with sleep. Be careful taking high doses of some of the energizing supplements discussed in this book since some of them, such as tyrosine, can cause a restless sleep even if taken in the morning. Their effect can also be additive when combined with caffeine.
4. Eating a small or moderate, late-night snack about one or two hours before bedtime may actually promote sleep, especially if the meal includes carbohydrates (such as bread, whole grains, legumes, fruits, potatoes, pasta, or rice).
5. Stop mental activity at least one hour before bed and allow your mind to switch to fun reading, or watching a comedy film or TV show. You could tape your favorite prime-time sitcom and

then watch it before bed. Watching a horror movie or a violent TV show is not a good idea. You may find some of the violent scenes incorporated into your dreams.

6. Use earplugs to muffle noises. You may be surprised how many noises can potentially disturb your sleep. These could be such interruptions as a dog barking, traffic, airplanes flying overhead, birds chirping outside your room in the early morning, or a noisy bed partner. Using earplugs has had a significant influence on my ability to get deep, uninterrupted sleep and has enormously influenced my daytime productivity.
7. Wear eyeshades to block the early-morning light. There is no reason to wake up earlier than you have to and then to try, unsuccessfully, to catch a few more minutes of shallow sleep.
8. Try one or more relaxation techniques when you get to bed. When lying on your back, shake and loosen a leg and foot. Take a few, slow, deep breaths by expanding your belly. Proceed to shake and loosen the other leg and foot and then return to your abdomen for a few more relaxed breaths. Proceed with this relaxation to your arms, shoulders, and neck. Now relax your facial muscles—especially the muscles around the eyes and mouth. Remember to return to your breath after relaxing each muscle group. Before you know it, you'll be drifting into a deep slumber.

Now that we've looked at the positive steps you can take to improve your mind naturally, in the next chapter let's examine some habits that interfere with optimal brain function.

SIX

Beware of Brain Busters

Marty is a fifty-four-year-old accountant who went through a difficult divorce after a twenty-two-year marriage. This chronic stress interfered with his performance at work. "I used to have a photographic memory, but now I have trouble remembering the names of some of my clients," he laments.

Denise, a forty-eight-year-old lawyer, was diagnosed with high blood pressure by her internist. She was prescribed propranolol, a medicine that slows heart rate and lowers blood pressure. However, about a month after starting this medicine, Denise noticed that she was not thinking as sharply and had difficulty recalling phone numbers.

Stress and certain medicines can interfere with optimal mental function. In this chapter, I will discuss several conditions that impede mental health, and provide suggestions on how to best deal with them.

STRESS, ANGER, AND ANXIETY

There's an intricate connection between the brain and the body. They communicate with each other through hormones, neurotransmitters, and many other types of chemical messengers. For instance, the hypothalamus and pituitary, two regions in the brain that control various hormone systems, respond immediately to stress by releasing hormones that stimulate the adrenal glands to release cortisol. Excess cortisol can wreak havoc with brain cells, interfering with mental functioning and memory. In turn, the immune system and some of the organs in the body release chemicals that pass into the brain and influence the function of brain cells.

Whether physical (e.g., intense athletic competition, illness) or psychological (e.g., emotional difficulties, financial worries), stress has definite harmful biological effects. Our immune system responds quickly to our thoughts and emotions. On the surface of white blood cells, there are receptors to which hormones and neurotransmitters attach. When we are under stress, substances released by the brain attach to the cells of the immune system and disturb their proper functioning. Positive thoughts and emotions are believed to enhance the immune system. The immune system can in turn send substances back to the brain, altering the release of neurotransmitters, thus influencing mood and cognition.

Consequences of excess stress include:

- **Immune system malfunction**, making us more susceptible to colds and various infections. Certain germs or immune cells fighting these germs can potentially cross the blood-brain barrier and damage brain cells. Lack of sleep significantly interferes with proper immune function.
- **Increased risk for heart disease, high blood pressure, and stroke**. Chronic damage to arteries leading to the brain can decrease blood flow to vital systems. There is a type of brain deterioration called "multi-infarct dementia" that occurs when frequent small clots travel to the brain and limit the blood supply to brain cells. Tiny strokes that go unnoticed can, over the long run, damage a number of areas in the brain. When enough damage occurs, noticeable signs of mental malfunction become ap-

parent. A large blood clot can cause a blockage of a major artery, incapacitating a wide segment of the brain, thus causing a major stroke.

- **A higher likelihood for chronic fatigue and various musculoskeletal aches and pains**. These chronic conditions can lead to low mood and can necessitate the use of painkillers that can have detrimental effects on brain function.

Luckily we can do something about stress by attempting to channel our thoughts to a more positive direction. Some of the stress we encounter is self-induced or self-aggravated, not necessarily due to external circumstances. Rather, it is due to our underdeveloped coping skills. While stuck in traffic, we can boil with frustration or we can turn on the radio and hum along with the songs. How we handle stress is often more important than the nature of the stress. Does every little thing throughout the day that doesn't go according to your plans upset you, or do you calmly adapt to unplanned situations?

The first step in dealing with stress is to identify its source. The next step is to take specific action to relieve or eliminate the source. Take a moment now or later to list any sources of stress in your life in a private journal. Beside each entry write down how you plan to deal with that stressor. There are times when life is cruel, and our load is so heavy, that we just want to sit and cry. That's perfectly okay. Crying helps to wash away toxic chemicals and hormones built up during stress, which in turn improves mood. It's healthy to cry once in a while.

There are many ways to relieve stress: vacations, playing with pets, improving sleep and physical health, finding satisfying work, consulting with an understanding friend or family member, establishing financial security, and participating in exercise, sports, yoga, prayer, or meditation.

If all of the above suggestions are not enough to relieve your stress, you can temporarily use certain natural supplements available over-the-counter to help you ease your tension. The two most effective ones are the herb kava and the nutrient 5-HTP, which converts into serotonin. The B vitamins are also very good in helping us build resistance to stress. Many other nutrients, such as methyl donors (Chapter 10), mind energizers (Chapter 12), and certain herbs such as ginseng can improve energy levels and well-being and hence make it easier to deal with everyday stress.

SMOKING

Elderly smokers experience a greater loss in the ability to think, perceive, and remember than people who have never smoked or who have quit smoking. The mental decline of elderly smokers may be tied to "silent strokes"—very small strokes that go unnoticed. Smoking is known to cause atherosclerosis, not just of the heart vessels, but also the vessels that supply blood and oxygen to the brain. In addition to damaging blood vessels, smoking causes constriction of arteries, clot formation, oxidation, and raised blood pressure. Smoking or exposure to cigarette smoke may also be linked to an increased risk of hearing loss.

ALCOHOL

Excess alcohol has a direct neurotoxic effect, meaning that it kills neurons. Excessive alcohol consumption also reduces the availability of certain B vitamins. One or two glasses of alcohol per day should not interfere with memory to any significant extent.

BE KIND TO YOUR MIND

Everything discussed in this book deals with improving mental health. In this section, I wish to further explain how we can make our minds even healthier by replacing negative input with positive input. As you know, whatever enters our stomach affects our body. We need to be as careful about what enters our mind. For instance, unhealthy relationships with parents, a spouse, a lover, relatives, an employer, or roommates can give the ego a regular beating. The constant exposure to this emotional insult inevitably has a detrimental influence on the psyche, and consequently affects physical and mental health. If improving the lines of communication and restoring healthy interactions are not possible, it may be appropriate to temporarily withdraw from unhealthy relationships and give time to heal.

Reduce your exposure to movies, books, and television programs that portray violence, horror, or negativity. Viewing violence may make some people, especially children and teenagers, more aggressive. Even if the violence does not manifest externally, violent programs can affect dreams. Radio and television shows that continually criticize and disparage individuals or groups due to ethnic, racial, and sexual orientation, are an additional source of negativity. Be conscious of what you feed your mind. Watching excessively violent movies, or reading similar books, is for the mind what consuming junk food is for the body.

If you're a news junkie, take breaks once in a while for at least a weekend and don't read a newspaper or watch the news on television.

COMMON MEDICAL CONDITIONS ASSOCIATED WITH COGNITIVE DECLINE

There are a number of medical conditions that can interfere with proper brain function.

Cardiovascular diseases, such as hypertension and coronary artery disease, are closely associated with brain function. The common pathway that leads to damage to the arteries in the rest of the body most likely also damages the arteries that supply the brain. Therefore, any lifestyle and dietary changes that you make to improve your cardiovascular health—such as exercise, relaxation, increasing whole-foods intake, and so on, will help circulation to the brain.

Common hormonal conditions that can influence brain function include diabetes and thyroid disease, particularly hypothyroidism. Make every effort to keep your blood sugar under control and see your physician regularly for exams to rule out any major problems with your thyroid gland and other organs.

The immune system is intricately involved in keeping the brain healthy. A number of immune compounds released by the body, such as interleukins, are able to cross the blood-brain barrier and influence neurons. Hence the healthier your immune system is, the healthier your brain.

Significant nutritional deficiencies are uncommon in this country, but there are large numbers of individuals, especially the elderly, who have marginal intakes of many nutrients. Hence, B-vitamin supplements and other nutrients can sometimes have a dramatic influence on brain health.

BRAIN-BUSTING MEDICINES

One of the most common causes of rapid cognitive decline is the use of certain prescription drugs.

Sedatives and sleeping pills often have immediate and dramatic effects on memory and clarity of thinking. Regular use of some of these drugs can sometimes cause irreversible memory impairment. The occasional use of melatonin is an alternative to sleeping pills, while kava and 5-HTP can substitute for antianxiety agents in the therapy of mild-to-moderate anxiety. Do not be concerned about the infrequent use of a pharmaceutical sedative: this should not interfere with memory.

Cholesterol-lowering drugs have become mainstays over the past five years, after several studies hinted they reduce the risk of dying from heart attacks. Millions of Americans now take a type of drug called statins. Although these drugs may reduce the risk of coronary artery disease in the short term, they may also have negative effects on mental cognition. Some studies have shown that those who lower their cholesterol levels excessively seem to have reduced mood, attention, and concentration, and are more likely to die by car accidents and suicide. Cholesterol is one of the important components of brain lipids. It plays a crucial role in the cell membrane, helps in the transmission of nerve signals, and serves as the precursor to the manufacture of pregnenolone, DHEA, estrogen, and all the other steroid hormones. By blocking the formation of cholesterol, or excessively lowering its concentration through drugs, are we also decreasing levels of steroid hormones in the brain? Could the shortage of these hormones in the brain lead to depression, memory loss, and cognitive decline? The answers are not yet available, but this possibility must be considered. Cholesterol-lowering drugs may be appropriate to use if cholesterol levels are very high, but keep in mind the negative influence these drugs may have on cognition. Make an attempt to lower your cholesterol through diet or natural supplements.

There are many other types of drugs that could interfere with cognition. These include certain beta-blockers, painkillers, calcium channel blockers, anticonvulsants, chemotherapeutic agents, and muscle relaxants. Ask your physician whether any of the medicines you are taking has a negative influence on the brain, and whether there may be better pharmaceutical or nutritional alternatives.

PART IV

A Practical Guide to Mind-Boosting Supplements

SEVEN

Mind Your Brain Fats

Doctors generally believe that the best way to treat mood, thought, and memory disorders is with pharmaceutical medicines that directly influence levels of brain chemicals such as serotonin, dopamine, and acetylcholine. Although drugs have very important clinical uses, they are only part of the solution. A comprehensive approach to treating cognitive disorders should include foods and supplements that benefit the overall health of brain cells.

One way to influence brain health dietarily is to consume the right fats and oils. About 60 percent of the brain consists of lipids (fats) which make up the lining, or cell membrane, of every brain cell. The types of fats present in the brain influence its structure and function. How well your mind works depends, in the long run, on what you eat.

This chapter will focus on fatty acids, particularly the omega-3s. Omega-3 oils are found mostly in fish and flaxseed, as well as sold in supplements sold over-the-counter.

WHAT COGNITIVE BENEFITS DO OMEGA-3 OILS HAVE?

Following are some of the improvements you may notice if your intake of omega-3s is currently low and you begin to consume more fish, or take fish-oil or flaxseed-oil supplements:

- Improved mood
- Enhanced clarity of thinking
- More serenity and mental stability
- Better concentration and focus
- Better vision

WHICH CLINICAL CONDITIONS CAN OMEGA-3s BENEFIT?

The clinical application of omega-3s is not yet well researched, but scientists have begun to explore the role of these important fats in the following conditions:

- Age-related cognitive decline
- Depression and bipolar disorders (manic depression)
- Anxiety disorders
- Addiction disorders
- Schizophrenia

It's quite possible some of these conditions will eventually be found to respond partially or significantly to supplementation with omega-3s.

DIETARY FATS AND THE BRAIN

Carolyn, a writer from Marina Del Rey, California, speaks for many when she says, "Fish oils make me more focused and serene. In addition, I get far less brain fatigue in the late afternoon." Marvin, a forty-three-year-old musician from New York, says, "I don't notice the effects from fish oils if I take a low dose. When I take more than 3 grams, I find that I have a sense of well-being and feel more aware." And Kevin, a twenty-eight-year-old actor from Los Angeles, adds, "Within a few hours of taking fish-oil capsules, I notice my vision to be improved. Colors are more vivid and everything is in better focus."

Changing the types and amounts of fats we consume can influence the fatty composition of brain cells and other cells in the body.

The lining of every cell in the body—for instance, the lining of red blood cells that carry oxygen—is made of fats. The type of fats in a red-blood-cell membrane can change very quickly, often within hours, based on the type of fats present in a meal. This change influences the fluidity of the cell membrane. The more fluid a red-blood-cell membrane, the easier it is for it to squeeze through tiny capillaries and supply oxygen and nutrients to remote areas of the body.

The fats that make up brain-cell membranes are much more resistant to changes in diet than the fats forming the cell membranes of other tissues in the body. The brain has developed an excellent ability to preserve its fatty composition despite shortages of essential fats in the diet. However, it is possible to alter the fat content of the brain through diet. We know this is true through animal studies. Manipulating the fatty-acid content of a rat's diet changes the fatty-acid composition of the brain-cell membrane within as brief a time period as three weeks (Yehuda 1998). The types of fats making up the cell membrane influence how well brain cells interact and communicate with each other. Since the membranes of brain cells can be influenced by dietary composition, our objective, then, is to consume the proper types of fats and oils, and in their proper balance, which will guarantee that neurons function at their best.

Before I discuss what kinds of fats and oils you should eat, and the proper amounts, let's review some of the basic chemistry of fats. This review will make it much easier to understand the importance of omega-3 oils in brain health, and it will also help you understand the role phospholipids play in cognition. (Phospholipids are discussed in Chapter 8.)

The ABCs of Fats and Oils

Lipids is a general term that includes fats, oils, cholesterol, and other substances that are fat-soluble. A simple difference between fats and oils is that fats are solid at room temperature, while oils are liquid. Fats and oils are triglycerides, which means they are made of a three-carbon molecule called **glycerol** attached to three long-chained carbon molecules called **fatty acids** (see Figure 7.1).

Figure 7.1—Basic Structure of a Fat or Oil

FATTY ACID——G

FATTY ACID——G

FATTY ACID——G

The three G's stand for the *glycerol molecule.*

There are dozens of common fatty acids present in the diet and the body. The length of these fatty acids varies, but most of them contain between four and twenty-four carbon atoms. Fatty acids are the building blocks for fats and oils, and are divided into two groups—saturated and unsaturated (see Figures 7.2 and 7.3).

Figure 7.2—Saturated Fatty Acid

C-C-C-C-C-C-C-C-C-C-C-C-C-C-C-C-COOH

Figure 7.3—Unsaturated Fatty Acid

C-C-C=C-C-C=C-C-C=C-C-C-C-C-C-C-C-COOH

Saturated fatty acids are found mostly in meat, animal fats, dairy products, lard, and some tropical oils. Each carbon atom in these saturated fatty acids is attached to two hydrogen atoms. In contrast, **unsaturated fatty acids** contain a double bond, meaning that two neighboring carbon atoms have each lost a hydrogen atom (Figure 7.3 shows a double bond as =): When fatty acids are unsaturated, they are more fluid and flexible. This is often a desirable trait.

Unsaturated fatty acids are in turn divided into two major groups:

1. **Monounsaturated** fatty acids are found in such vegetables as olives and avocados. They have one double bond. *Mono*, as you may know, means "one."
2. **Polyunsaturated** fatty acids have two or more double bonds. *Poly* means "many." The more double bonds present, the more fluid the fatty acid. You can generally tell the degree of unsaturation of a particular food by how fluid it is in the refrigerator or at room temperature. For instance, cheese contains mostly saturated fats, and is hard. Olive oil is monounsaturated and stays relatively liquid at room temperature, but hardens in the refrigerator. Fish oils and polyunsaturated oils, such as canola, can stay fluid even in very cold temperatures.

Many polyunsaturated fatty acids, called **nonessential fatty acids**, can be manufactured by the body. Others, called **essential fatty acids**, must be ingested through foods. There are two types of essential fatty acids: omega-3s and omega-6s.

A) **Omega-3** fatty acids are made from a fatty acid called *alpha-linolenic acid* (ALA) (see Figure 7.4). *Omega* is the last letter in the Greek alphabet. In naming fatty acids, the last carbon of the chain is called *omega*. The fatty acid shown in Figure 7.3 is an omega-3 fatty acid since one of the double bonds starts on the third carbon from the left. ALA is found predominantly in flaxseed oil (also known as linseed) and hemp-seed oil. Green leafy vegetables, soybeans, walnuts, and canola oil have small amounts of omega-3 fatty acids. Omega-3 fatty acids are beneficial because they provide fluidity to cell membranes and improve communication between brain cells. Omega-3s also reduce the clotting ability of platelets, thus potentially decreasing the incidence of heart attacks and strokes. Two very important omega-3 fatty acids are eicosapentanoic acid (EPA) and docosahexanoic acid (DHA). They are found in seafood, especially mackerel, salmon, striped bass, rainbow trout, halibut, tuna, and sardines. Supplements of fish oils that contain EPA and DHA are sold over-the-counter. DHA is also sold by itself. In the body, DHA is found mostly in the brain, retina, and in sperm. DHA plays an important role in vision.

B) **Omega-6** fatty acids are made from *linoleic acid*, a fatty acid found in vegetable oils such as corn, safflower, cottonseed, and sunflower. Mayonnaise and salad oils normally contain a great amount of omega-6 fatty acids. As you can see in Figure 7.5, linoleic acid is eventually converted into arachidonic acid (AA), a beneficial fatty acid that, in excess, can induce inflammation, clotting, and have other unhealthy actions. Unlike omega-3s, which are concentrated in the brain, omega-6s are found in most tissues in the body. The double bond of an omega-6 fatty acid starts six carbons from the left. Most Americans generally have a much higher intake of the omega-6s than the omega-3s.

Up to 50 percent of the fatty acids in the gray matter in the brain is made of DHA and AA.

Figure 7.4—The Making of Omega-3s

Alpha-linolenic acid (ALA) has 18 carbon atoms and 3 unsaturated bonds

▼

Eicosapentanoic acid (EPA) has 20 carbon atoms and 5 unsaturated bonds

▼

Docosahexanoic acid (DHA) has 22 carbon atoms and 6 unsaturated bonds

The mineral zinc, and other vitamins and minerals, help convert EPA to DHA. DHA has the ability to convert back into EPA (Hansen 1998). The human body is not able to make omega-3s from omega-6s, or vice versa.

Figure 7.5—The Making of Omega-6s

Linoleic acid (LA) has 18 carbon atoms and 2 unsaturated bonds

▼

Arachidonic acid (AA) has 20 carbon atoms and 4 unsaturated bonds

The body uses omega-3s and omega-6s to produce several types of important substances such as prostaglandins, eicosanoids, and leukotrienes. These substances have a number of effects on the brain and body. They can act as hormones, are involved in the immune system, blood-pressure control, clotting, heart rhythm, and they even influence tumor inhibition or formation. The types of fatty acids in the diet is known to influence the release of hormones by the pituitary gland.

Fats to Shun

Trans-fatty acids are new forms of fats that have been introduced over the past few decades. These are chemically altered and twisted fatty acids that are unhealthy and are not easily used by the body. Trans-fatty acids are generally found in margarine and many processed foods, pastries, donuts, corn chips, and processed cereals. Any type of fatty acid can be damaged and become harmful to the body if deep-fried. **Hydrogenated fats and oils,** commonly found in processed foods, are also unhealthy. Hydrogenation means adding hydrogen atoms, thus transforming a fatty acid from unsaturated to saturated.

A full explanation of fats can be quite complicated. I have listed several books in the bibliography that can give you a more detailed explanation. In this chapter it has been my goal to simply give you some background on the chemistry of these fatty acids in order to discuss the enormous importance of omega-3 oils to body and brain health.

Fish Oils and Mood

Over the past few years, scientists have attempted to determine whether the types of fats we consume have an influence on mental function. It appears that there is a connection. Drs. Joseph Hibbeln and Norman Salem Jr., from the National Institute of Alcohol Abuse in Rockville, Maryland, have done epidemiological studies to determine this connection. In an article published in *Lancet* in 1998, the doctors compare fish consumption to the prevalence of major depression in eleven countries. They found that the more fish consumed in a country, the less the risk for depression. The doctors say, "Increasing rates of depression in the last century may be influenced by the consumption of increased amounts of saturated fatty acids and omega-6 fatty acids and the decreased consumption of omega-3 fatty acids."

Studies indicate that DHA levels in red-blood-cell membranes are low in those who are depressed (Peet 1998). No studies have yet been published to determine if supplementing with fish oils leads to mood elevation, but these oils have been found to play a role in the relief of manic-depression.

Manic-Depression

Also known as "bipolar disorder," patients with this condition go through cycles of feeling mania (euphoria, racing thoughts, hyperactivity) followed by cycles of depression. The standard pharmaceutical approach to treating bipolar disorders is with lithium or drugs such as valproate and carbamazepine. Dr. Andrew Stoll, M.D., from the Department of Psychiatry at Harvard Medical School, has tested fish oils on this condition. He conducted a four-month double-blind placebo-controlled study using about 10 grams a day of concentrated fish oils. Overall, nine out of fourteen patients responded positively to fish oils, compared to three out of sixteen patients receiving a placebo. Dr. Stoll tells me, "In cases of mild bipolar disorder, it would be worthwhile to first try a therapeutic approach with fish oils before proceeding to pharmacological therapy."

Interestingly, Dr. Stoll reports that a preliminary study using flaxseed oil with fifty patients showed that ALA, the fatty acid found in flax, has mild mood-stabilizing and antidepressant effects.

Help for Schizophrenia?

Even relatively difficult mental conditions such as schizophrenia may partially be influenced by the fatty acid content in the brain. In a study done at the Northern General Hospital in Sheffield, England, dietary supplementation for six weeks with 10 grams per day of concentrated fish oil led to significant improvement in patients with schizophrenic symptoms (Laugharne 1996).

Malcolm Peet, M.D., a professor at Northern General Hospital, has found that supplementation with fish oils as an addition to existing antipsychotic drug treatment leads to significant improvement in treatment-resistant schizophrenic patients. Interestingly, when he compared the effectiveness of EPA versus DHA, he found that EPA was very effective, while DHA wasn't. (Most fish-oil capsules contain both EPA and DHA, but supplements are now available that contain only DHA.) This result was unexpected since, unlike DHA, EPA is not found in significant amounts in the brain. One can speculate that perhaps EPA is better transported through the blood-brain barrier than DHA, or perhaps EPA influences a set of immune and hormonal reactions that DHA does not. EPA can be converted into DHA which then is incorporated into cell membranes.

Fish Oils and Learning

Although long-term human studies have not yet been conducted evaluating therapy with fish oils and cognitive function, a one-year study in mice gives us some preliminary answers (Suzuki 1998). Adult mice were fed a regular diet that included either 5 percent palm oil (containing mostly a 16-carbon saturated acid) or 5 percent sardine oil. At the end of the year, it was determined that the mice taking the sardine oil had a higher brain concentration of DHA. Their synapses and cell membranes were more fluid, and their maze-learning ability was better than the mice that were fed palm oil.

Seeing Is Believing

The rods and cones of the retina in the eyes are very rich in DHA. Hence, a deficiency in dietary fish oils will reduce the photoreceptor activity of retinal cells, and thus reduce visual acuity. On the other hand, supplementation with fish oils (or flaxseed oil) could lead to visual improvement with enhanced color perception.

Since levels of DHA in the brain decline with age, it is likely that the levels of DHA also decline in the retina. Is it possible that daily intake of fish oils can improve vision in older individuals? Hopefully future research can give us some answers. Chapter 20 discusses in more detail the effects of omega-3 oils and various nutrients on vision.

The Author's Experience

I have taken fish oils off and on for many years. I've experimented with very high daily dosages in order to determine if these oils have any immediate effects. The highest daily dose I have taken is thirty capsules, each containing 300 mg of a combination EPA and DHA, totaling 9,000 mg. I took this dose in the morning, and by late afternoon I noticed the onset of clarity in vision, with objects looking sharper and clearer. There was a slight improvement in distance vision, and details became more noticeable. Fine print became easier to read. The visual improvements continued and improved on subsequent days when I kept taking between ten to twenty capsules. Fish-oil supplementation also makes me more serene, focused, and balanced. The effects, though, are subtle. I currently take about 600 to 1,200 mg of EPA/DHA per day except on days when I eat fish.

My experience with flaxseed oil has also been positive. When I take a tablespoon or more, I find that I have more energy and clarity of vision. This seems to improve over the following days if I continue taking the flaxseed oil. At higher doses, such as two tablespoons, I become overstimulated and experience insomnia.

THE SIMPLE "BRAIN FOOD" PLAN

Dietary intake of omega-3 fatty acids varies significantly in the North American population. As a rule, most Americans have a low intake of fish oils, perhaps as low as 200 mg per day of EPA and DHA. In cultures where fish is a large part of the diet, such as Eskimo or Japanese, the intake of fish oils can approximate 3 to 10 grams a day (one gram equals 1,000 mg).

For optimal brain function, I recommend that you consume fish at least two or three times a week. If your diet does not include enough of the omega-3 fatty acids or enough fish, you could consider taking supplements of fish oils or flaxseed oil. Vegetarians, or those who don't eat fish, are good candidates for taking omega-3 supplements. As a rule, ingesting about half a gram to 2 grams of a combination of EPA and DHA daily should be sufficient.

There are dozens of different brands of fish-oil capsules sold in health-food stores, pharmacies, and retail outlets. Each of them is likely to contain a different amount of EPA and DHA, but generally each capsule contains between 200 to 400 mg of a combination EPA and DHA. There are even small, fruit-flavored capsules for children. Fish oils are best stored in the refrigerator.

For many years fish-oil supplements were available as a combination of EPA and DHA. Recently, DHA has been made available by itself. This algae-derived product does not contain EPA, but has 100 mg of DHA per capsule. A DHA capsule is much more expensive than a standard fish-oil capsule. The question arises as to whether DHA has benefits over that of fish oils. I had a discussion about this matter with Artemis Simopoulos, M.D., an expert on omega-3 oils, and President for the Center for Genetics, Nutrition, and Health in Washington, D.C. She tells me, "If someone were to take fish-oil supplements, I do not see a need to take DHA supplements alone instead of fish-oil supplements that contain both EPA and DHA."

Based on all the information available to date, it appears that taking a DHA supplement by itself may not be necessary. For now, I recommend to my patients that their supplements include a combination of EPA and DHA. Taking the combination is much cheaper than taking DHA by itself. It's possible, though, that future research may indicate that DHA alone may be helpful in infants, the elderly, in pregnancy, or other conditions. Algae-derived DHA supplements are also an option for strict vegetarians who do not wish to ingest fish oils.

Flax or Fish?

Since the fatty acid ALA in flax oil can convert into EPA and DHA, why not just take flaxseed oil supplements instead of fish oils? This could well be a good option for those who prefer flaxseed over fish oils. However, it is possible that some people may not have the adequate biochemical ability to convert ALA into EPA and DHA. The conversion is a difficult process and may require more than 10 grams of ALA to make 600 mg of EPA or 400 mg of DHA (Gerster 1998). Lloyd Horrocks, Ph.D., Professor Emeritus of Medical Biochemistry at Ohio State University in Columbus, Ohio, is an expert on fish oils. He says, "The enzymes that convert shorter-chain and less-saturated fatty acids such as ALA into the longer-chain EPA and DHA may not work efficiently in everyone."

It has also been suggested that several conditions or situations may lead to inadequate activity of the enzymes that convert ALA to EPA and DHA (Drevon 1992). These conditions include aging, diabetes, intake of trans-fatty acids, and a large intake of saturated fatty acids.

Norman Salem Jr., Ph.D., at the National Institutes of Health, tells me,

> Our research team has been studying omega-3 fatty-acid metabolism in humans. Our conclusion is that the conversion of ALA to DHA in most adults is adequate to maintain DHA status in

the brain, but may not be adequate in newborns or individuals with certain metabolic disorders. A poorer DHA status associated with aging may occur due to dietary changes in essential fat, as well as low levels of antioxidant intake. We do know that the intake of omega-3 fatty acids is deficient in the Western diet. Most individuals are overdosing on *safflower, corn,* and *peanut oils.* These should be replaced by *canola, flaxseed,* and *olive oils.* In addition, it is important to consume the longer-chain omega-3 fats found in foods like fish and perhaps poultry. If chickens are fed foods high in long-chain fatty acids, the eggs will contain a higher proportion of these fatty acids. With time, eggs from better-fed chickens should become more widely available to consumers.

Based on the evidence currently available, it appears that most adults are able to convert flaxseed oil to EPA and DHA, but there could be some individuals unable to do so adequately. This could be due to genetics, medical conditions, excessive dietary intake of saturated or trans-fatty acids, or the aging process. Therefore, just to be on the safe side, it would seem reasonable to include flax oil in the diet, yet also eat fish or take fish-oil supplements. This way, all essential omega-3 fatty acids such as ALA, EPA, and DHA, would be ingested.

Cautions and Side Effects

There are few drawbacks in supplementing with omega-3 oils. However, due to the fact that these oils can thin the blood, it is possible that very high doses could increase the risk of bleeding. If a bleed occurs in the brain, it is called a hemorrhagic stroke. *The incidence of bleeds is rare, but could be of clinical significance if a person is already taking high doses of aspirin, coumadin, or other blood thinners.* The incidence of a hemorrhagic stroke is significantly less compared to the potential benefits from the reduction in heart attacks and strokes due to blood clots.

Recommendations

Individuals with a low intake of seafood or foods supplying omega-3 fatty acids are likely to benefit from supplementation with fish oils or flaxseed oil.

At this point, it is difficult to give precise dosages of EPA and DHA that would apply to everyone. Individuals may vary in their requirement for these fatty acids, depending on their dietary intake and their biochemical ability to convert smaller-chain omega-3s to EPA and DHA. As a rule, eating fish two or three times a week supplies about seven grams of EPA/DHA per week. A reasonable approach for someone who does not eat fish is to supplement with about one gram of a DHA/EPA combination on a daily basis. However, some individuals may require much higher doses to notice positive effects or to treat certain psychological, neurological, or medical conditions.

EPA and DHA are important fatty acids in maintaining proper memory and cognitive function. Therefore, I consider fish oils to be a crucial component of the mind-boosting program presented in this book. Taking a small amount of antioxidants, such as a few units of vitamin E, along with the fish-oil supplements seems prudent.

Over the next few years we may discover that omega-3–oil supplements have a positive influence on a number of neurological or psychiatric conditions. The influence in some cases may be minor, but even a small benefit would be worthwhile since fish oils or flaxseed oils are inexpensive and do not have major side effects, as do some pharmaceutical drugs.

EIGHT

Memory Boosters—Phospholipids, Choline, and Related Nutrients

Like omega-3 fatty acids, phospholipids are also important for optimal brain health. As the name implies, phospholipids are made of the combination of lipids (fats) and the mineral phosphorus. Phospholipids are found in high concentrations in the lining of practically every cell of the body, including brain cells. They help brain cells communicate, and influence how well receptors function. Although present in many foods, phospholipids are found in higher concentrations in soy, eggs, and the brain tissue of animals. There may actually be a biochemical rationale for the folk wisdom that eating brain makes one smarter.

The two most common phospholipid supplements sold over-the-counter are phosphatidylcholine (PC) and phosphatidylserine (PS). Phosphatidylcholine is also known as lecithin. This chapter explains the role and function of phospholipids, their clinical effects, and practical recommendations for or against supplementation.

In addition to these phospholipids, I will also discuss choline, a nutrient that helps form phosphatidylcholine. Acetylcholine, the brain chemical involved with memory, is made from choline. Choline has been sold over-the-counter for many years. A new and more activated

WHAT BENEFITS DO CHOLINE AND PHOSPHOLIPIDS PROVIDE?

Individuals who don't have a good dietary intake of phospholipids may find that taking these nutrients leads to an improvement in learning and memory. Most young and healthy people who take PS or PC are not likely to notice any significant changes, although supplements could help some seniors. The effects from choline and its cousin, CDP-choline, are more noticeable.

WHICH CONDITIONS CAN CHOLINE AND PHOSPHOLIPIDS BENEFIT?

The clinical application of these nutrients has not yet been fully evaluated, but scientists have studied their role in age-related cognitive decline (ARCD), Alzheimer's disease, and Parkinson's disease. No firm conclusions are available yet as to whether PS and PC help improve these conditions. Choline and CDP-choline could potentially be beneficial in ARCD and Alzheimer's disease.

form of choline, called CDP-choline, became available in the United States in 1998.

PHOSPHOLIPIDS AND HEALTHY CELL MEMBRANES

A lining called the "cell membrane" surrounds each brain cell. Without a healthy cell membrane, we cannot have optimum memory and mental function. Phospholipids play several roles in the brain. They not only determine which minerals, nutrients, and drugs go in and out of the cell, but also influence communication between brain cells by influencing the shape of receptors and promoting the growth of dendrites.

Since phospholipids help form the cell membrane of the trillions of cells in the body, it makes sense that they would have an influence not just on the brain, but also on a number of organs and tissues, including the heart, blood cells, and the immune system. As we age, there's a decline in the amount of phospholipids making up cell membranes (Soderberg 1991).

The Making of Phospholipids

Phospholipids are compounds made of two fatty acids attached to glycerol, the mineral phosphorus, and an amine. An amine is a molecule that has nitrogen attached to a few carbon atoms. The two most common fatty acids attached to phospholipids in the brain are DHA and arachidonic acid (AA). You may recall from Chapter 7 that DHA is found in fish oils.

Phosphatidylcholine (PC) is the most abundant phospholipid in brain-cell membranes, comprising about 30 percent of the total phospholipid content, while phosphatidylserine (PS) makes up less than 10 percent.

The fatty-acid content of brain phospholipids can be altered by the composition of the diet, particularly just before and after birth, and the phospholipid composition of the brain can be manipulated even in adults. Animal studies have indicated that omega-3 fatty acids added to the diet of rats are able to travel to the brain-cell membranes and become part of the phospholipids (Jumpsen 1997). If one's diet includes seafood, then there will be an adequate amount of DHA present in the phospholipids forming the cell membrane of neurons.

The fatty-acid composition of phospholipids can deteriorate with aging and disease. As we age, many of the long-chained polyunsaturated fatty acids, such as DHA, can become shortened and more saturated. This can interfere with the optimal functioning of neurons.

In order to better understand how the nutrients in this chapter work, it helps to know how they are related to each other. As you can see from Figure 8.1, PS can be converted into PC; choline converts into CDP-choline and then PC.

All of the nutrients listed in this figure, except for acetylcholine, are available over-the-counter as supplements. Acetylcholine is a brain chemical involved in memory and learning, among various other functions.

Figure 8.1—Relation of Choline to Acetylcholine and Phospholipids

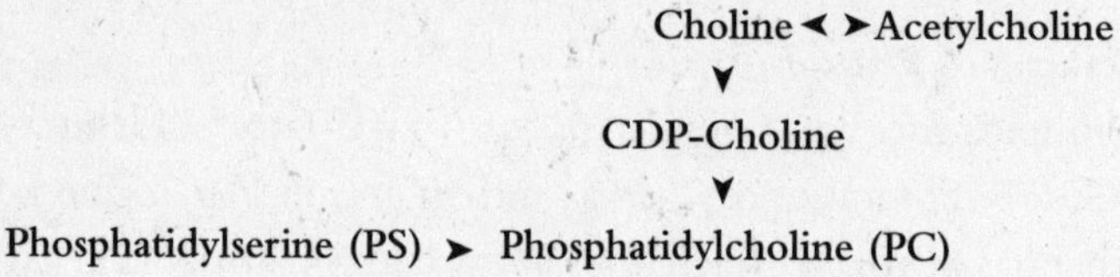

Choline ◀ ▶ Acetylcholine

▼

CDP-Choline

▼

Phosphatidylserine (PS) ▶ Phosphatidylcholine (PC)

Having presented the overview, let's now discuss specific nutrients and the research evaluating their role in the therapy of cognitive disorders.

CHOLINE

Choline helps form phosphatidylcholine, the primary phospholipid of cell membranes. Choline also helps form acetylcholine, one of the important brain chemicals involved in memory. This nutrient, usually as part of phosphatidylcholine, is widely available in a number of foods, particularly eggs, fish, legumes, nuts, and meats and vegetables, as well as in human breast milk. Dietary intake of choline ranges from 300 to 900 mg a day. Most individuals who have a normal diet are not deficient in choline. The importance of choline was emphasized in 1998 when the National Academy of Sciences classified it as an essential nutrient. In the past, it was thought that the human body made adequate amounts when needed. However, a study by Dr. Steven Zeisel, from the Department of Nutrition at the University of North Carolina at Chapel Hill, demonstrated that volunteers on a choline-deficient diet were not able to produce enough of this nutrient (Zeisel 1991).

According to the results of several studies in rats, providing choline during pregnancy enhances memory and learning capacity in the fetus

(Williams 1998). Dr. Christina Williams, a behavioral neuroscientist at Duke University in Durham, North Carolina, says her study findings demonstrate "that supplementation with choline during the last third of pregnancy has fairly dramatic and long-lasting effects on the memory of offspring."

Several studies have been done administering choline to humans in order to evaluate memory function. The results have been mixed, with some showing positive results (Sitaran 1978) while others indicate no improvement (Mohs 1980).

Choline has also been tested in bipolar disorder, also known as manic-depression. When six patients already on lithium were given choline bitartrate, five of them had a substantial reduction in manic symptoms (Stoll 1996).

A 1997 study published in *Advances in Pediatrics* by Dr. Zeisel showed that choline reserves are depleted during pregnancy and lactation (Zeisel 1997). This depletion may affect normal brain development and memory in the offspring. The National Academy of Sciences suggests that pregnant women consume at least 450 milligrams of choline per day.

Availability and Dosage

Choline is sold in vitamin stores in doses ranging from 250 to 500 mg, and in a number of forms including choline bitartrate, choline chloride, and choline citrate.

The Author's Experience

Within a few hours of taking choline, I notice an improvement in focus that lasts most of the day. I have not experienced side effects with dosages smaller than 500 mg. On a dosage of 1,500 mg, I experienced increased body warmth.

Cautions and Side Effects

A high intake of choline is associated with mild gastrointestinal distress, nausea, sweating, and loss of appetite (Wood 1982).

Recommendations

Individuals whose diet includes a wide variety of foods are not likely to suffer from choline deficiency. Growing infants, pregnant or lactating women, and individuals with liver cirrhosis may be deficient in choline (Zeisel 1994). Whether choline supplements benefit older individuals with age-related memory decline has not yet been adequately determined. Because of its relative safety and potential benefits, I recommend small amounts of choline for the elderly who have age-related cognitive decline (see Chapter 18 for specific recommendations). Choline can be taken occasionally by younger individuals on days when better concentration and focus would be helpful.

CDP-CHOLINE

CDP-choline stands for cytidine 5-diphosphocholine. This nutrient is approved in Europe and Japan for use in stroke, Parkinson's disease, and other neurological disorders (Secades 1995). In a way, you could consider CDP-choline as a more potent form of choline. Studies show that CDP-choline helps make phosphatidylcholine (PC) in human brain-cell membranes in older individuals (Babb 1996); may increase acetylcholine synthesis; improves mental performance in patients with Alzheimer's disease when given at a daily dose of 1000 mg per day (Cacabelos 1996); and even improves memory in elderly patients with memory deficits (Alvarez 1997). A Belgian study has shown that administrating CDP-choline to dogs improves their ability to learn and remember (Bruhwyler 1998).

Dr. Vittorio Porciatti at the Institute of Neurophysiology in Pisa, Italy, tells me,

> CDP-choline is commercially produced in Europe under several product names. Neurologists have found this nutrient useful in Parkinson's disease, brain trauma, and aging in general. It may surprise you that I mention Parkinson's disease. In addition to

> the understandable action on cell membranes, we have been somehow surprised that CDP-choline has dopamine-like effects. Interestingly, dopaminergic-like activity seems to be long-lasting, possibly due to stabilization of the effects at membrane level. We have found no significant side effects with CDP-choline even for long therapy cycles. In one study we gave a dosage of 1 gram a day for fifteen days to young individuals. They reported improvement in visual clarity. (Porciatti 1998)

Availability and Dosage

CDP-choline became available over-the-counter in the U.S. in 1998, but it's expensive and not widely distributed. Most pills come in a 250 mg dose.

The Author's Experience

Within an hour of taking a 250 mg CDP-choline pill on an empty stomach, I notice being more alert and motivated. The effects last a few hours. In addition, colors seem brighter and sharper, and occasionally I have noticed a slight libido enhancement. Because of the alertness it produces, I have difficulty sleeping if I take this nutrient in late afternoon or early evening.

Cautions and Side Effects

Toxicology studies show that CDP-choline is safe and produces no serious side effects in doses ranging from 500 to 1,000 mg a day (Secades 1995). However, most of the studies lasted less than a few weeks. *Long-term safety is not known.*

Recommendations

CDP-choline has been used successfully in Europe for many years, but clinical experience in the U.S. is limited. This nutrient appears to have a more direct and immediate effect on the brain than its cousin choline. However, it is difficult to predict at this time the long-term benefits or risks of regular use.

CDP-choline is a promising nutrient and I suspect that with time it will become more popular. Eventually we may find a role for it in the therapy of certain neurological conditions such as Alzheimer's disease, and perhaps Parkinson's disease. Combining choline, lecithin, and CDP-choline for therapeutic purposes is an interesting concept which has not yet been formally tested.

PHOSPHATIDYLCHOLINE (LECITHIN)

Lecithin is also known as phosphatidylcholine (PC), although lecithin is also a term loosely applied to describe a combination of PC with other phospholipids. Most people normally ingest 3 to 6 grams of lecithin a day through eggs, soy, and meats. Vegetables, fruits, and grains contain very little lecithin.

PC is the most abundant phospholipid component in all cells, and PC levels in brain-cell membranes decline with age.

Several studies have been done with PC to investigate its effects on memory. The results of the studies have not been consistent. Some have shown positive responses (Sorgatz 1987, Ladd 1993), while others showed no difference in memory or learning after lecithin administration (Gillin 1980).

Lecithin has even been evaluated in Parkinson's disease (Tweedy 1982). In this nine-week-long double-blind study, sixteen elderly patients took a daily dose of approximately 32 grams of a commercial lecithin preparation. Marked clinical improvement was not observed, but there was a slight improvement in memory, cognition, and motility.

Availability and Dosage

Lecithin is sold in the form of liquid, capsules, or granules. The amount of PC in each product varies between different brands. The lecithin you buy in a health-food store will generally include about 10 to 70 percent PC, along with other lipids. Different types of lecithin will differ in their lipid compositions depending on the source of the lecithin—soy or egg yolk—or the extraction process.

The Author's Experience

I have interviewed many individuals who have taken lecithin in order to improve cognition. The reports have not been impressive. The majority of users do not notice any obvious benefits from lecithin.

Lecithin does not provide me with cognitive effects. I have taken fifteen capsules a day of lecithin for a week without a noticeable effect on alertness, vision, or mood. Each capsule contained 1,200 mg of PC.

Recommendations

Research findings regarding the role of PC in cognition have not been consistent. My professional and personal experience with PC does not indicate that this supplement has any dramatic effects on mental abilities. Based on the available evidence, it appears that the cognitive benefits of taking lecithin are likely to be minor.

As a rule, individuals who consume a wide variety of foods are not likely to suffer from PC deficiency. Whether lecithin supplements benefit a subgroup of seniors with age-related memory decline has not yet been adequately determined. It is certainly possible that there are those who may have a biochemical difficulty in making adequate amounts of PC and would benefit from additional supplementation.

If you are planning to take lecithin, keep your dosages low, such as 3 grams a day or less.

PHOSPHATIDYLSERINE (PS)

Although lecithin (PC) has been available as a supplement for many decades, PS became available to the North American market in the mid-1990s. In the past, PS was obtained from the brains of cows. In fact, if you read some of the research studies published on PS, it will identify this nutrient as BC-PS. The BC stands for "bovine cortex," or cow brain. The reason BC-PS is not sold is because of the fear of viruses or infectious agents being inadvertently introduced in the PS product when extracted from the brains of cows. The PS currently available over-the-counter is derived from soy.

Several studies have evaluated the role of oral administration of BC-PS in both animals and humans. In general, the results have shown positive benefits. However, we need to keep a very important point in mind. The studies with PS have used bovine cortex as the source. Can we assume that the results with soy-derived PS would be similar? Each PS molecule contains two fatty acids. The fatty acids in PS derived from soy are mostly 16- and 18-carbon molecules such as palmitic, oleic, linoleic, and linolenic acids. These are small-chain fatty acids and have fewer double bonds than the fatty acids in PS derived from bovine brains, such as arachidonic acid and DHA, which are polyunsaturated and have longer chains of 20 and 22 carbons.

Human studies with soy-derived PS have not been published in reliable, peer-reviewed journals. However, there have been a number of studies evaluating the role of BC-PS in cognitive function, particularly in age-associated memory impairment and Alzheimer's disease. Most of these studies have indicated that BC-PS improves memory and cognition in those with age-related cognitive decline (Crook 1991, Cenacchi 1993), and helps improve memory and recall in patients with Alzheimer's disease (Engel 1992, Crook 1992).

Companies promoting soy-PS make positive claims about this supplement and defend its promotion by citing research studies done on BC-PS. I interviewed many experts on fats, including Drs. Simopoulos, Horrocks, Schmidt, Hibbeln, and Salem, regarding their opinions on PS. All experts were unanimous in their assessment that one can't automatically use the studies done with BC-PS to claim soy-PS provides the same benefits.

Dr. Arjan Blokland and colleagues, from the Brain & Behavior Institute in Maastricht, The Netherlands, investigated the cognition-enhancing properties of different types of PS in rats. Seventeen-month-old rats were treated daily for four weeks with a dose of 15mg/kg of PS derived from bovine cortex (BC-PS), soybeans (S-PS), egg (E-PS), or placebo. (The PS was administered by injection into the abdominal cavity, whereas in humans PS is ingested orally. A dose of 15 mg/kg is equivalent, by weight ratio, to about a 1,000 mg daily dose in humans.) It appeared that the cognition-enhancing effects of S-PS were not different from those of BC-PS, although E-PS did not produce any improvement in cognition. The authors concluded, "On the basis of the present study, it was concluded that S-PS, but not E-PS, may have comparable effects on cognition when compared with BC-PS.

I interviewed Dr. Blokland regarding his findings. He told me,

> In our research group we have had lively discussions regarding the blood-brain barrier crossing of PS. Some of my colleagues did not believe that this molecule could pass the BBB. They assumed that the fatty acids first had to be removed [in the gastrointestinal system or bloodstream] from the rest of the molecule in order to enter the brain, and in the brain fatty acids were again connected to the serine group. But others did not agree. Our human psychopharmacology unit also conducted a study with PS but did not find a positive effect on cognitive performance (unpublished data). They suggested that the PS was metabolized too rapidly and that not enough PS entered the brain. We are now planning an actual study in which we would like to apply radio-labeled PS in order to determine the activity of the labeled PS in the membrane fraction of rat brain tissue. That should answer our questions.
>
> It is unclear to us why egg PS showed inactivity, whereas soy PS was active. Given the fact that the fatty acid composition of egg PS (relatively high in arachidonic acid and docosahexaenoic acid) matches more closely the composition of brain phospholipids compared to soy PS, which is high in linoleic acid, we were surprised by this observation. We can therefore only spec-

ulate that the egg PS may have lost bioactivity because of the breakdown of the bioactive compound during processing or storage. We were surprised by this finding but we do not have a clue for this behavioral observation.

Availability and Dosage

BC-PS is not available in the United States, but soy-derived PS is sold in vitamin stores. Each 500 mg gel capsule contains several phospholipids, with 100 mg being actual PS. PS is an expensive nutrient; each pill costs between 50 cents and one dollar. Again, it is worth emphasizing that the PS currently available is derived from soy products and thus has a different fatty-acid composition and chemical makeup than the bovine cortex–derived PS used in published studies.

The Author's Experience

I interviewed thirty individuals who have taken PS. The majority did not notice an effect from this nutrient while a minority reported minimal benefits in alertness and memory. Overall, the results were not impressive.

I have taken soy-derived PS in dosages ranging from 100 to 1,400 mg. I do not notice an effect when taking a dosage less than 300 mg. With higher amounts, I've noticed a mild enhancement in alertness, concentration, and focus, which can persist late into the evening. No visual changes were apparent. On the downside, I had a slight feeling of malaise and my mood was lower. In my experience, the short-term effects from soy-PS are not as dramatic as choline and some of the other nutrients discussed in this book. Perhaps an older person who is lacking PS in his or her brain-cell membranes may notice the effects of PS more clearly.

Cautions and Side Effects

Short-term human studies have found few side effects from supplemental intake of PS. *The long-term effects are not known.* It's possible that PS could influence, positively or negatively, the immune system, the function of red blood cells, or have other effects. PS is found in the inner cell membrane of red blood cells and is involved in the process of blood-clotting. We don't know whether excess intake of PS will alter red-blood-cell membranes and increase the propensity for clots.

One Japanese study raises a concern (Uchida 1998). Cells removed from Chinese hamster ovaries were incubated with PS and other phospholipids such as PC. The cells exposed to PS became damaged, shrank, and died, while those exposed to the other phospholipids were not affected. The clinical significance of this in vitro study, if any, is currently not known.

Recommendations

Many human studies have shown BC-PS to have benefits in the therapy of cognitive impairment. No human trials with soy-derived PS have been published in peer-reviewed journals.

As to the effectiveness of soy-PS compared to BS-PC, I agree with the experts cited above that it is not scientifically acceptable to make claims regarding benefits of soy-PS using the results obtained with BC-PS.

Since we only have soy-PS available over-the-counter, one interesting option is to take fish-oil capsules along with it. This way it's possible we may more closely mimic the results of the studies done with BC-PS. Dr. Hibbeln says, "Available data in both rodents and in cell culture indicate that the rate of PS synthesis depends on the availability of DHA." However, whether taking fish oils along with PS will be advantageous is difficult to predict.

We need several studies published with soy-PS before we have a better grasp of its clinical uses. I don't yet have a firm opinion on whether the potential benefits of soy-PS supplementation justify its cost. Most young and middle-aged individuals who have a good diet that includes eggs, soy, and other sources of phospholipids, and omega-3 oils, will not need additional PS. However, it's possible that a subgroup of older patients with age-related cognitive decline might potentially benefit from PS supplements.

With the availability of choline, CDP-choline, PC, and PS, how do you decide which ones to choose? Unfortunately, not enough research is yet available to provide firm recommendations.

Of the four nutrients discussed in this chapter, I've personally noticed the clearest immediate effects from choline and CDP-choline. However, it is difficult to predict which of these nutrients provides the best long-term benefits with the least risk. Noticing an immediate effect from a nutrient does not mean that it is the best choice for long-term therapy.

Many of the nutrients discussed in this chapter could well have overlapping physiological functions and effects. One approach is to try each one separately to determine which one(s) provide the clearest benefit.

NINE

Mood and Energy Lifters—B Vitamins and Coenzymes

A B-vitamin supplement is the cheapest, safest, and most reliable way to improve your well-being and overall mental ability. I recommend the Bs to those who wish to improve their mood, mental clarity, and energy. The effects of the B vitamins are subtle, especially in the young who normally have adequate dietary intake of these nutrients. Improvements in cognitive functions from the B vitamins are particularly noticeable in middle-aged individuals and the elderly.

In addition to discussing the B vitamins, this chapter will review coenzymes—the new, more activated forms of the B vitamins—and make recommendations on how to reduce levels of homocysteine, an amino acid derivative that can be harmful to the cardiovascular and neurological system when present in excess.

THE Bs IN THE BRAIN GET AN A

B vitamins help in energy production, and deficiencies lead to fatigue and poor mental functioning. The increased consumption of refined foods has decreased the amounts of B vitamins present in our diet.

BENEFITS OF B VITAMINS

Since B vitamins and their coenzymes play important metabolic roles in numerous biochemical reactions throughout the body, they can influence just about every aspect of brain and physical health. As a rule, individuals who take B vitamins notice improvements in

- Mood and energy
- Alertness
- Learning and memory
- Speed of thinking
- Verbal fluency
- Concentration and focus
- Visual clarity

WHICH CLINICAL CONDITIONS DO THE Bs BENEFIT?

Because of their wide range of effects, B vitamins and their coenzymes can potentially be helpful in

- Depression
- Age-related cognitive decline
- Anxiety disorders
- Addiction disorders
- Chronic fatigue
- Alzheimer's disease
- Parkinson's disease

However, on the positive note, small amounts of B vitamins are regularly added to some food products, such as cereals.

The question of whether B-vitamin supplementation is necessary in healthy individuals who have a normal diet has been debated ever since vitamins were discovered. The results of several studies over the past few years have influenced my decision in favor of low-dose supplementation. There can be cognitive improvements from taking B vitamins. Back in 1995, Dr. David Benton and colleagues from the University College Swansea, in Great Britain, gave ten times the recommended daily allowance of nine vitamins (mostly the B vitamins) to healthy college students (Benton 1995). The study lasted for one year. The students reported improvement in mood and feeling more agreeable. There was also an improvement in cognitive functioning, especially in regards to concentration. Many of my patients consistently report that B-vitamin supplementation improves their energy, concentration, and mood while helping them handle everyday stress better.

For otherwise healthy individuals, supplementation with one to three times the recommended daily allowance of the B vitamins is suggested. Higher dosages may be required for individuals with medical, psychiatric, or neurological disorders.

UNDERSTANDING COENZYMES

In the past few years, many of the B vitamins have become available in their more activated forms known as **coenzymes**. For instance, the B-vitamin niacin is now available in a coenzyme form known as NADH. An enzyme is basically a protein that promotes chemical changes in other substances, itself remaining unchanged in the process. A coenzyme is a substance that facilitates or is necessary for the action of an enzyme.

The brain, just like a car, needs fuel. Our primary source of fuel is through fats, proteins, and carbohydrates in the diet. After digestion in the stomach, foodstuffs are absorbed into the bloodstream and circulate to various tissues and cells where they are broken down into even smaller particles. One of these particles is a two-carbon molecule known as acetyl. Enzymes help break down these fats, proteins, and carbohydrates into acetyl, and they then help extract the final energy from acetyl through a process called the Krebs cycle, named after the German biochemist who defined it. This energy is in the form of ATP (adenosine triphosphate). Enzymes also need helpers, and these helpers are called coenzymes. Most of the coenzymes in the body are partly made from vitamins, such as vitamins E, C, lipoic acid, and riboflavin (vitamin B_2).

The coenzyme form of a B vitamin often has a significantly more powerful effect than a regular B vitamin. The coenzyme forms of the B vitamins are an exiting addition to the field of nutrition. It is quite possible that the elderly or certain individuals with a particular biochemical deficiency may not be able to make adequate amounts of the coenzyme forms of the B vitamins despite adequate intakes of the individual B vitamins. Hence the coenzyme forms should be seriously considered as a supplement in those who do not respond to the regular B vitamins. Some companies include most of the Bs in their coenzyme form together in one pill. I think these products deserve serious consideration, especially for their use in the middle-aged and the elderly.

The Individual B Vitamins and Their Coenzymes

Thiamin (B_1) is necessary for the metabolism of carbohydrates and amino acids to adenosine triphosphate (ATP), the primary source of energy in the human body. Thiamin is found in good amounts in milk, lean pork, legumes, rice bran, and the germ of cereal grains, but is lost during food processing and cooking. The current recommended daily allowance (RDA) by government advisory panels is about 1.5 mg.

Studies indicate that supplementation with thiamin provides cognitive benefits. Dr. Benton and colleagues gave 50 mg of thiamin daily to young adult females for a period of two months (Benton 1997). The women reported being more clearheaded, composed, and energetic. The taking of thiamin had no influence on memory, but reaction times were faster following supplementation. Prior to taking the thiamin, the women had normal blood levels of this vitamin.

Researchers at Princess Margaret Hospital in Christchurch, New

Zealand, measured thiamin levels in elderly individuals before giving them 10 mg of the vitamin a day (Wilkinson 1997). Only the subjects with low thiamin concentrations showed benefits. They had an improvement in quality of life, with more energy and deeper sleep, along with decreased blood pressure and weight.

Thiamin is now also sold in its coenzyme form, called cocarboxylase or thiamin pyrophosphate (TPP). Human studies giving TPP to evaluate cognitive functioning have not yet been published.

Riboflavin (B_2) is a yellow-colored nutrient involved in dozens of metabolic pathways leading to energy production and the making of fatty acids and sterols. Good sources are lean meats, eggs, milk, some vegetables, and enriched cereals. The recommended daily intake is about 1.5 mg. You may notice your urine turning a deeper-yellow color after taking riboflavin.

Riboflavin is part of two larger activated coenzymes known as flavin adenine dinucleotide (FAD) and flavin mononucleotide (FMN). FMN is now available as a supplement. One product contains 25 mg of FMN per pill. Human studies giving FAD or FMN in order to evaluate cognitive functioning have not yet been published.

Niacin (B_3), also known as nicotinamide and nicotinic acid, plays essential roles in a large number of energy pathways. Perhaps as many as 200 enzymes are dependent on this nutrient.

Nicotinamide is part of the coenzyme known as nicotinamide adenine dinucleotide (NADH), which itself is sold as a supplement. I will discuss NADH later in this chapter since several studies have been published regarding this coenzyme. Good sources of niacin are meats, legumes, fish, and some nuts and cereals. The recommended daily intake is about 15 to 20 mg.

Pantothenic acid (B_5) is essential for biological reactions involving acetylation and energy production. This vitamin helps in the formation of acetylcholine, the metabolism of fatty acids, and the incorporation of fatty acids into cell-membrane phospholipids. Pantothenic acid is also involved in making steroid hormones, vitamin A, vitamin D, and cholesterol. Good sources are egg yolk and fresh vegetables. The recommended daily intake is about 5 mg. Pantothenic acid is sold over-the-counter in dosages ranging from 5 to 250 mg.

My patients report that pantothenic acid helps improve their mood and energy. Personally, I notice an improvement in alertness, concentration, energy, and visual clarity with dosages ranging from 100 to 250 mg. I do experience insomnia, though, when I take more than 250 mg, even if I take it in the morning. Benita von Klingspor, a nutritionist in Marina Del Rey, California, says,

> Pantothenic acid is one of my favorite nutrients. I know the effects of this nutrient extremely well, since I've been taking 100 to 250 mg most mornings for more than thirty years. I often recommend it to many clients with low energy. Pantothenic acid increases their alertness and focus, improves their mood, and enhances their joy in life. They begin to have more interest in whatever they're doing. However, if people take too much pantothenic acid, they can become overstimulated, wired, and easily aggravated.

Pantothenic acid is available in its activated form, known as pantethine. Pantethine, itself, is part of coenzyme A, a very important substance that participates in the metabolism of carbohydrates, amino acids, fatty acids, and dozens of other important chemical reactions. Cognitive effects of oral administration of pantethine to humans have not been published. Pantethene is sold over-the-counter in doses ranging from 5 to 50 mg. In my experience, a lower dosage of *pantethine* provides similar effects as a higher dosage of *pantothenic acid*.

Pyridoxine (B_6), also known as pyridoxal, is widely available in most foods including vegetables, legumes, nuts, seeds, and animal products. The coenzyme form of pyridoxine is pyridoxal phosphate (PLP), and at least 100 different metabolic reactions are helped by PLP. PLP is a necessary coenzyme in the production of brain chemicals: It helps the conversion of 5-HTP into serotonin, tyrosine into dopamine and norepinephrine, and the production of other neurotransmitters such as histamine and GABA. The recommended daily intake is about 1.5 mg. Deficiencies in B_6 can lead to low mood.

Human studies with PLP in mood disorders and depression have not yet been published. PLP is available in pills ranging from 5 to 20 mg. Some individuals notice the difference between regular B_6 and the coenzyme form. Joan, a fifty-three-year old patient from Beverly Hills, California, says, "I've taken good-quality B vitamins for a few years. Recently I tried the pyridoxal phosphate form of B_6. It really has increased my energy, mood, and alertness."

Folic acid, also known as **folate**, generally functions in cooperation with vitamin B_{12} in many metabolic reactions, including the synthesis of DNA. Folic acid helps reduce levels of homocysteine, a substance that can increase the risk for atherosclerosis (discussed later in this chapter). This vitamin functions as a methyl donor (see Chapter 10). Folic acid is found in almost all foods, and the recommended daily intake is about 400 micrograms. The coenzyme form of folate is called tetrahydrofolate.

Cobalamin (B_{12}), or cyanocobalamin, has a number of important roles in metabolism, including the synthesis of DNA. This function is particularly crucial when it comes to making new red blood cells. Hence, a deficiency of B_{12} leads to anemia. The formation of myelin—the white sheath surrounding nerves—is partly dependent on B_{12}. Deficiencies in B_{12} intake lead to nerve damage, memory loss, poor coordination, low mood, and mental slowness. This nutrient, along with folic acid and B_6, helps to lower levels of homocysteine. High homocysteine levels are suspected to be one of the factors causing hardening of the arteries.

The recommended daily intake of B_{12} is about 3 micrograms, but much higher dosages are well tolerated. B_{12} is found mostly in meats and fish. Vegetarians can become deficient in this vitamin if they don't take supplements. B_{12} deficiency can occur in the elderly due to malabsorption from the intestinal tract. If you have gastritis, absorption problems, autoimmune disorders, insulin-dependent diabetes, certain thyroid disorders, or take antacids or other medicines that reduce stomach acid, you could have problems maintaining adequate B_{12} levels. Hence, a monthly B_{12} shot, in a dose of 1 mg (1,000 micrograms), could well provide you with positive cognitive benefits. Sublingual forms of B_{12} are also available (which dissolve under the tongue).

There are two coenzyme forms of B_{12}, adenosylcobalamin and methylcobalamin. Adenosylcobalamin is sold over-the-counter as dibencozide, in a dose of 10,000 micrograms (10 mg), which is a large dose. Human studies evaluating its role in cognitive disorders have not been published. It's quite possible that with age, nutritional deficiencies, or enzyme deficiencies, some individuals may not be able to convert B_{12} into its coenzyme forms.

Biotin is involved in the metabolism of carbohydrates and fats. It is widely available in foods, particularly egg yolk, soybeans, cereal, legumes, and nuts. Bacteria in the gastrointestinal system also make it. The RDA ranges from 30 to 100 micrograms.

Recommendations

All of the B vitamins are important, and supplementation would probably benefit most everyone. For healthy individuals, taking one to three times the RDA of the Bs would be sufficient. You will find B complex supplements that say "B-50" or "B-100" on the label. This means that many of the B vitamins, such as thiamin and riboflavin, are found in dosages of 50 or 100 mg per pill. The RDA for thiamin and riboflavin is about 1.5 mg. The average, healthy person does not need to take these high dosages. However, biochemical individuality certainly does exist. Dr. David Benton, Ph.D., who researches the influence of B vitamins on cognition, says, "There can be enormous differences in the needs of vitamins. It wouldn't be unusual for some individuals requiring twenty times the amount of a particular vitamin compared to others in a similar age group."

Part V has recommendations on B-vitamin dosages for different age groups, and Part VI has dosage suggestions for those with mood disorders, Alzheimer's disease, or Parkinson's disease.

NADH (NICOTINAMIDE ADENINE DINUCLEOTIDE)

I remember my high-school biology class where I first tried to learn the complicated Krebs cycle and how energy in the form of ATP was derived from sugars, amino acids, and fats. I did recall coming across NADH (nicotinamide adenine dinucleotide), a coenzyme that helps in this complicated process of energy extraction. Although NADH is only one of the B-vitamin coenzymes discussed earlier in this chapter, it has been studied more thoroughly than the other coenzymes. NADH has been promoted very heavily through ads and magazine articles ever since it was introduced to the health industry in the mid-1990s.

One of the functions of NADH is to help convert the amino acid tyrosine into the important brain chemical dopamine. Dopamine is involved in mood, energy, sexual drive, concentration, memory, and muscle movement. NADH may also regenerate the antioxidant glutathione (see Chapter 11). NADH is normally found in meat, fish, and poultry. The content of NADH in fruits and vegetables is negligible.

Most users report NADH improves mood, energy, vision, alertness, and sexual interest. Mark, a fifty-six-year-old accountant from Oakland, California, likes NADH. He says, "I have been taking 2.5 mg of NADH three times a week for the last few months, and my brain's working again. I can think clearer and sharper." Shelly, from Mission Viejo, California, reports that "NADH makes me more alert and provides a sense of well-being. I currently take it about once a week."

According to Georg Birkmayer, M.D., an Austrian researcher whose family has been instrumental in developing a trademarked NADH product, "NADH energizes both body and brain activity, improves alertness, concentration, emotion, drive, and overall mood enhancement." Dr. Birkmayer goes on to say that no adverse or side effects have been reported with NADH. He further claims that NADH improves memory, slows the aging process, and is helpful in a variety of conditions including Alzheimer's disease, Parkinson's disease, chronic fatigue syndrome, depression, and overall lack of energy.

Are any of these claims true?

A small number of short-term studies done with NADH have shown that NADH has slight-to-moderate benefits in regards to depression, Parkinson's disease, and Alzheimer's disease (Birkmayer 1991, 1993, and 1996). An eight-week double-blind study done at Georgetown University Medical Center found some patients with chronic fatigue syndrome to benefit from taking NADH at a daily dose of 10 mg (Forsyth 1998). However, long-term studies are required to determine if benefits from taking daily NADH continue with time, or whether tolerance develops.

Availability and Dosage

Most of the NADH pills come in doses of 2.5 and 5 mg. Individually sealed, airtight pills are a good option. One of the shortcomings with NADH is its cost, which can be close to a dollar a pill.

NADH is best taken in the morning, generally on an empty stomach. Alertness and mental clarity are often noticed within a few hours. Be careful when using multiple supplements that increase energy since their effects can be cumulative and lead to overstimulation.

The Author's Experience

Does NADH really improve energy, concentration, and mood? I have taken NADH on numerous occasions. Within an hour or two of swallowing a pill on an empty stomach in the morning, I notice an increase in alertness, feelings of well-being, vitality, visual clarity, and sexual interest. The effects last most of the day. However, I do develop a tolerance to NADH if I take it regularly.

Cautions and Side Effects

Reports of untoward effects from the use of a 2.5 mg dose of NADH are infrequent. Higher doses can sometimes lead to insomnia, anxiety, fatigue, and overstimulation. George, a forty-two-year-old lawyer from Philadelphia, says, "I like the 2.5 mg dose of NADH because of the alertness it provides. However, when I take 5 mg or more, it makes me too stimulated, almost with a panicky feeling." As more individuals start taking NADH, we may come across additional reports of side effects.

The risk of side effects increases when NADH is combined with other stimulants. A few patients have found that high dosages used daily for prolonged periods led to mood swings, anxiety, and sleeplessness which resolved when the NADH was stopped. Until we learn more about the long-term effects of NADH, I do not recommend its use on a daily basis for prolonged periods.

One user noticed that NADH helped her chronic fatigue, but things didn't go well when she stopped. Betty, a thirty-six-year-old homemaker from Houston, says, "I have chronic fatigue syndrome [CFS], and was taking 10 mg of NADH daily. I know it really helped my energy level and mood. But I began to have stomach upset from it and stopped for a few days. I then fell quickly into a very bad CFS 'crash,' the worst one in months." I recommended that Betty only take 2.5 mg of NADH every other day.

Recommendations

Studies with NADH have been short and therefore it is difficult to give definitive recommendations on its long-term benefits. Could side effects develop that we are not currently aware of? It is unlikely that NADH by itself will be the magic bullet in Parkinson's disease, Alzheimer's disease, chronic fatigue syndrome, and other conditions. However, if longer-term studies do confirm some of the minor benefits reported in preliminary findings, NADH could be an additional supplement doctors can recommend in the fight against certain chronic neurological diseases. And NADH, along with other B-vitamin coenzymes, could well be useful in age-related cognitive decline.

If you plan to take NADH on a regular basis, I would recommend you limit your frequency to no more than three times a week. Please keep in mind, though, that the other B vitamins are also very important.

B VITAMINS AND HOMOCYSTEINE

Homocysteine is a derivative of the amino acid methionine. It received a great deal of media attention in 1997 following publication of articles in medical journals indicating that a high blood level of homocysteine is a potential risk factor for atherosclerosis and heart disease. Kilmer McCully, M.D., a pathologist at the Veterans Affairs Medical Center in Providence, Rhode Island, had been claiming for at least two decades that homocysteine is as important a risk factor for heart disease as cholesterol, but few in the medical profession paid serious attention to his claim. Dr. McCully was vindicated with the publication of additional scientific articles in the 1990s, most of which confirmed the dangers of elevated homocysteine levels. Fortunately, homocysteine levels can be easily lowered by taking supplements of B vitamins, particularly folic acid, B_6, and B_{12} (see Figure 9.1).

In addition to contributing to cardiovascular conditions, homocysteine may also be detrimental to the brain since it can act as a toxin to brain cells. Dr. Lucilla Parnetti and colleagues, from Perugia University in Italy, published in article discussing the role of homocysteine in cognitive decline (Parnetti 1997). They say, "Homocysteine may represent a metabolic link in the cause of atherosclerotic vascular diseases and old-age dementias. Excessive homocysteine is an independent risk factor for coronary artery disease, peripheral vascular disease, and cerebrovascular disease. Homocysteine is a reliable marker of vitamin B_{12} deficiency, a common condition in the elderly, which is known to induce neurological deficits including cognitive impairment. A high prevalence of folate deficiency has been reported in geriatric patients suffering from depression and dementia. Both these vitamins occupy a key position in the remethylation and synthesis of S-adenosyl-methionine (SAMe), a major methyl donor in the central nervous system. Therefore, deficiencies in either of these vitamins leads to a decrease in SAMe and an increase in homocysteine, which can be critical in the aging brain." (I discuss SAMe in Chapter 10.)

Adequate intakes of folic acid, B_6, and B_{12} will assure that homocysteine levels are kept low. Considering the possibility that there may be individuals, especially the elderly, who are deficient in B_6, folic acid, and B_{12}, an inexpensive and simple way to decrease the rate of damage to the brain from homocysteine would be by supplementing with these vitamins (Woodside 1998).

Figure 9.1—The Role of B Vitamins in Homocysteine Metabolism

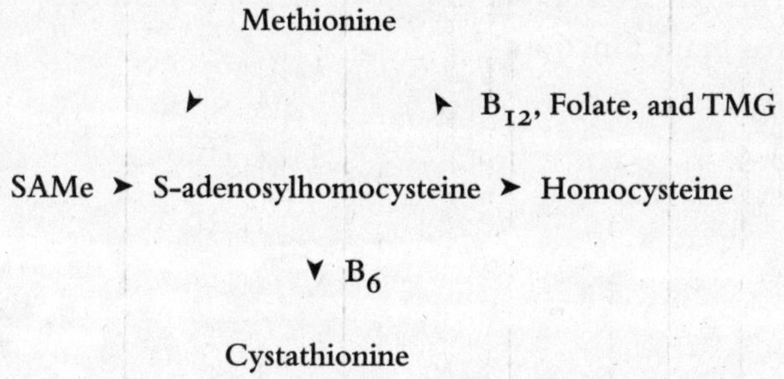

Methionine

➤ ➤ **B_{12}, Folate, and TMG**

SAMe ➤ S-adenosylhomocysteine ➤ Homocysteine

➤ **B_6**

Cystathionine

Nutritionists at Tufts University in Boston have also found a connection between B vitamins, homocysteine, and memory. They investigated the relationship between blood concentrations of homocysteine and vitamins B_{12}, B_6, and folate, and scores from a battery of cognitive tests for seventy male subjects, 54 to 81 years old (Riggs 1996). Lower concentrations of vitamin B_{12} and folate and higher concentrations of homocysteine were associated with poorer memory.

Summary

Because of the important role of each of the B vitamins in brain function, it makes sense that they should all be consumed as a group instead of taking large amounts of one or two. As a general guideline, it would be reasonable to take a supplement providing at least one to three times the RDA for these vitamins. Perhaps higher doses could be even more beneficial in certain individuals. A multivitamin bottle will list on the label the percentage of the RDA (or PDV—percent daily value) contained for each of the different vitamins. Let's say the RDA for thiamin is 1.5 mg. A reasonable dosage for the pills you buy could be anywhere between 1 and 5 mg. Make sure that the B vitamins contained in the pill are balanced and that you are not consuming large doses of a few while getting little or none of the others.

An exciting development over the past few years has been the introduction of the coenzyme form of the vitamins. It will take more research to evaluate many of these coenzymes and to determine who will best benefit from them and how they can be ideally combined for optimal brain function.

TEN

Methyl Donors—For More Energy, Better Mood (and Longer Life?)

Unless your major is college was chemistry, chances are you don't remember learning about **methyl donors**. But if you find the field of brain nutrients and anti-aging interesting, you will certainly want to learn more about these supplements. A methyl donor is simply any substance that can transfer a methyl group (a carbon atom attached to three hydrogen atoms [CH3]) to another substance. Many important biochemical processes rely on **methylation**, including the metabolism of lipids and DNA. Scientists suspect that adequate methylation of DNA can prevent the expression of harmful genes, such as cancer genes. It's quite likely that our body's ability to methylate declines with age, contributing to the aging process; therefore, supplementation could well be beneficial. The research in this area is still very new, and no firm answers are yet available. But one scientist is quite enthusiastic about methyl donors. Craig Cooney, Ph.D., Research Assistant Professor at University of Arkansas for Medical Sciences, Little Rock, Arkansas, is an expert on methylation and the author of scientific articles and a book on this topic. "I've been taking 250 mg of TMG a day since 1991," he says. "In my opinion, methyl donors have the potential to slow the aging process."

In the preceding chapter I mentioned that two of the B vitamins,

WHAT CAN METHYL DONORS DO FOR YOU?

Methyl donors help in the production of several brain chemicals and hence improve mood, energy, well-being, alertness, concentration, and visual clarity. A few people notice enhanced sexual enjoyment.

WHAT CONDITIONS CAN METHYL DONORS BENEFIT?

Methyl donors may be helpful in age-related cognitive decline, Alzheimer's disease, fighting depression, and overall health maintenance. They may perhaps also be helpful in Parkinson's disease.

folic acid and B_{12}, are also methyl donors. This chapter discusses four additional nutrients involved in methylation: TMG, DMG, SAMe, and DMAE. All but SAMe have been sold over-the-counter for a number of years. SAMe became available in the U.S. in 1996. Interestingly, some vegetables, such as onions, garlic, and beets, contain methyl donors (McCully 1997).

TMG (TRIMETHYLGLYCINE) AND DMG (DIMETHYLGLYCINE)

Trimethylglycine, or TMG, also known as betaine, is basically the amino acid glycine attached to three methyl groups. Dimethylglycine (DMG) is similar to trimethylglycine, except it has two methyl groups. You may recall that a "methyl group" is a carbon attached to three hydrogen atoms (CH3). Both of these nutrients are powerful methyl donors. Methylation is an important factor in many biochemical processes in the human body. In Chapter 9 I mentioned that the B vitamins folic acid and B_{12} lower levels of homocysteine, the harmful amino acid–like substance in blood which can cause hardening of the arteries, and possibly damage brain cells. By reducing homocysteine levels, the risk for heart disease can be reduced; TMG and DMG are also known to reduce homocysteine levels and therefore could be helpful in reducing the rate of heart disease. It's possible that as we age, the process of methylation becomes less effective, and supplementation with TMG or DMG may provide health and anti-aging benefits.

Methyl donors are also involved in the making of brain chemicals, which accounts for their cognitive effects. My clinical experience confirms that both TMG and DMG improve mood and energy. Brian, a twenty-nine-year-old laboratory technician from Torrance, California, speaks for many when he says, "TMG gives me more energy and clearer thinking. There's a sense of well-being that comes on that lasts all day." Paul Frankel, Ph.D., coauthor with Fred Madsen, Ph.D., of a book on methylation, says,

> I've been taking TMG since 1995 at a dose of 250 mg a day. Through my interviews with individuals who have taken TMG, I have come across many who report benefits—sleeping better, having more energy, and experiencing less chronic fatigue. TMG could also jump-start some people and help them fight their depression. A woman whose daughter was suffering with depression told me, "TMG gave me my daughter back."

Dr. Madsen adds, "I have taken TMG for more than ten years without any side effects. People who take TMG report that their mood is enhanced."

Availability and Dosage

TMG and DMG are sold in doses ranging from 100 to 500 mg. Beets, broccoli, and shellfish are good food sources of TMG. In fact, the source of most of the TMG sold over-the-counter is often from the sugar beet. Some DMG products are available in sublingual form, which are dissolved under the tongue, for a quicker onset.

The Author's Experience

I definitely notice a sense of well-being, alertness, and mental sharpness from either TMG and DMG, generally at doses between 100 and 500 mg. One morning I took three 750 mg pills of TMG (totaling 2,250 mg) on an empty stomach with an ounce of fruit juice just to see if there were any side effects. An hour later I felt the onset of mild nausea. Drinking a few ounces of milk relieved the nausea. As the day progressed, I felt more energetic and realized that my mood was enhanced. In the evening I took my routine three-mile walk and noticed that I had a great deal of energy. I kept walking and ended up covering twice my normal distance. The drawback was that at bedtime I was still alert and couldn't sleep at all. I got out of bed several times throughout the night. I continued feeling the alertness well into the morning of the next day. Apparently 2,250 mg is a very high dose and can have effects on the brain lasting more than twenty-four hours. A positive effect from taking DMG or TMG that I hadn't expected was an enhancement in libido. When I take a sublingual form of DMG, I notice the onset of alertness within thirty minutes.

Cautions and Side Effects

TMG and DMG, if taken in high doses, can cause nausea, restlessness, and insomnia along with elevated body temperature. According to Dr. Frankel, an additional side effect of high dosage can include muscle-tension headache.

I recommend not exceeding 250 mg of TMG or DMG or a combination on a daily basis until more is known about these supplements; dose of TMG and DMG should be reduced if you are taking B vitamins, SAMe, DMAE, or choline since all of these nutrients have overlapping functions.

Recommendations

TMG and DMG are underutilized nutrients that hold a great deal of promise, but unfortunately, few doctors are familiar with these nutrients. At this time, the clinical uses of TMG and DMG are not well defined, and whether they would be helpful in therapy for Alzheimer's and Parkinson's disease is not known. Since the body's ability to methylate declines with age, supplements of TMG or DMG in small amounts, such as 50 to 100 mg a day, may benefit middle-aged and older individuals.

SAMe (S-ADENOSYL-METHIONINE)

SAMe, a compound made from the amino acid methionine, is a methyl donor involved in the synthesis of dozens of important compounds in the body. SAMe has been available by prescription in Europe for many years as an antidepressant but has been available over-the-counter in the U.S. only since about 1996. Dr. Ascanio Polimeni, a physician in Rome, Italy, says, "SAMe is a wonderful supplement. Some doctors prescribe it in Europe as therapy for many conditions, including depression, chronic fatigue syndrome, and fibromyalgia. I have not found it to have any toxic effects even when I've prescribed it for several months in a row."

Unlike other methyl donors, where the research is scarce, there have been a number of studies with SAMe. These studies have shown that SAMe influences brain chemicals by helping to convert norepinephrine to epinephrine, and serotonin to melatonin; helping to make creatine, an important energy reservoir in muscle tissue; and helping to preserve glutathione, an important antioxidant. Furthermore, SAMe is involved in the formation of myelin, the white sheath that surrounds nerve cells and can improve the brain-cell membrane fluidity, thus potentially enhancing the function of receptors (Cestaro 1994).

SAMe and Mood

Because of its role in making neurotransmitters, SAMe has been tested in treating depression. A number of studies have been published, mostly in Europe, evaluating this nutrient's role in mood disorders. Back in 1994, Dr. G. M. Bressa, from the University Cattolica Sacro Cuore School of Medicine, in Rome, Italy, conducted a meta-analysis of the studies on SAMe (Bressa 1994). A meta-analysis is a statistical pooling of already-published research papers. Dr. Bressa concludes, "The efficacy of SAMe in treating depressive syndromes and disorders is superior to that of placebo and comparable to that of standard tricyclic antidepressants. Since SAMe is a naturally occurring compound with relatively few side effects, it is a potentially important treatment for depression."

The influence of SAMe on depression has also been tested in the United States. Back in 1994, researchers at the University of California Irvine Medical Center did a double-blind randomized trial involving a total of twenty-six patients (Bell 1994). They compared oral SAMe with oral desipramine (a pharmaceutical antidepressant). At the end of the four-week trial, 62 percent of the patients treated with SAMe and 50 percent of the patients treated with desipramine had significantly improved.

SAMe has even been tested in depressed postmenopausal women. Researchers from the University of La Sapienza in Rome, Italy, gave 1600 mg of SAMe for thirty days to eighty women between the ages of 45 and 59 who had experienced depression following either natural menopause or hysterectomy (Salmaggi 1993). There was a significantly greater improvement in depressive symptoms in the group treated with SAMe compared to the placebo group. Side effects were mild and transient.

Availability and Dosage

A major drawback to the use of SAMe is the expense. The retail price of SAMe is about a dollar per 200-mg pill. The suggested dose of SAMe to treat depression ranges from 100 to 400 mg a day. Many nutrients work in a fashion similar to SAMe, particularly other methyl donors such as DMAE (discussed below), TMG, DMG, and also some of the B vitamins. In fact, B_{12} and folate help the body produce SAMe. Therefore, your dosage of SAMe should be reduced if you are taking other methyl donors.

The Author's Experience

I started with two 200-mg pills of SAMe one morning at nine A.M. on an empty stomach and within an hour and a half noticed an increase in concentration, energy, alertness, and feelings of well-being. At eleven A.M. I took another 200-mg pill, and shortly thereafter ate my first meal of the day. An hour later, the alertness increased and my vision become slightly clearer. The sense of relaxed well-being continued all day and evening.

The highest dosage of SAMe I have taken is 800 mg, with no significant side effects.

Cautions and Side Effects

Dr. Polimeni has extensive experience with this nutrient. He says, "I have prescribed SAMe for depression for many years. This nutrient is safe, but high dosages can cause dry mouth, nausea, restlessness, and insomnia."

Kilmer McCully, M.D., from Veterans Affairs Medical Center in Providence, Rhode Island, has been researching homocysteine and methyl donors for the last three decades. He says, "High homocysteine levels can negatively influence cognitive decline. SAMe helps reduce homocysteine levels, and everything that I've read about it in scientific papers over the past three decades indicates that it is safe and beneficial. We know that SAMe levels decline with aging, and perhaps replacement in older age may prove to be advantageous."

Recommendations

SAMe has good potential to become a useful therapeutic agent for depression and age-related cognitive decline. Long-term studies are needed with SAMe before making widespread recommendations for its use. However, short-term human studies thus far have found it to be safe and effective. A major drawback to the long-term use of SAMe is its cost. Keep in mind, though, that TMG and DMG are also powerful methyl donors; they work in a similar fashion, and are cheaper.

Could TMG or DMG, taken along with B vitamins, offer benefits similar to SAMe's at a fraction of the cost? It is known that TMG can help to regenerate SAMe (Barak 1996). Dr. A. Barak and colleagues from the Department of Veterans Affairs Medical Center, in Omaha, Nebraska, say, "In view of the fact that SAMe has already been used successfully in the treatment of human maladies, TMG, being a SAMe generator, may become a promising therapeutic agent and a possible alternative to expensive SAMe."

A lot more research has to be done with SAMe to confirm some of the preliminary findings listed above. Dr. Bottiglieri and colleagues, from Baylor Research Institute, in Dallas, Texas, published a review article on SAMe and other methyl donors (Teodoro Bottiglieri 1994). They summarize,

> SAMe is required in numerous methylation reactions involving nucleic acids, proteins, phospholipids, amines, and other neurotransmitters. The synthesis of SAMe is intimately linked with folate and vitamin B_{12} metabolism, and deficiencies of both these vitamins have been found to reduce central-nervous system SAMe concentrations. Both folate and vitamin B_{12} deficiency may cause similar neurological and psychiatric disturbances including depression, dementia, and peripheral neuropathy. Studies support a current theory that impaired methylation may occur by different mechanisms in several neurological and psychiatric disorders.

DMAE (DIMETHYL-AMINO-ETHANOL)

Known chemically as dimethyl-amino-ethanol, DMAE has been known in Europe by the product name Deanol for more than three decades. DMAE has two methyl groups and is chemically similar to choline. This nutrient has been popular for many years among those interested in improving mental alertness and clarity of thinking.

Studies on DMAE go back to the 1950s. One double-blind, placebo-controlled trial performed on twenty-seven patients with severe Alzheimer's disease did not show any significant benefits (Fisman 1981). Another study on twenty-one patients with memory deficits was also discouraging since no improvement was found in memory (Caffarra 1980). However, DMAE was found to be helpful in patients with age-related cognitive decline. This nutrient was given in a dose of up to 600 mg three times a day for four weeks to fourteen older patients (Ferris 1977). Ten patients improved, and four were unchanged. The patients on DMAE had reduced depression, less anxiety, and increased motivation, but they had no improvement in memory. The researchers say, "The results thus suggest that although DMAE may not improve memory, it may produce positive behavioral changes in some senile patients." Dementia is a term that is now substituted for senility and is sometimes used to denote a severe case of age-related cognitive decline.

As you can see, limited studies with DMAE have not shown it to be effective on Alzheimer's disease or to help memory; however, DMAE does seem to help improve mood and motivation in older patients with dementia.

Availability and Dosage

DMAE is usually sold by the name of "DMAE bitartrate." A 350-mg pill of DMAE bitartrate yields 130 mg of actual DMAE. It is also available as liquid; one product contains 35 mg of DMAE per drop. Most users notice an effect from a dose of 100 to 200 mg of actual DMAE.

Users' Experiences

Audrey, a thirty-two-year-old patient from Hollywood, California, says, "I took a 350-mg pill of DMAE bitartrate at one P.M. By three P.M. I noticed a sharpened attention to detail, and a keener interest in observing my environment. DMAE definitely stimulated my thinking."

Most patients usually report similar effects, including the ability to focus better. However, higher doses can be counterproductive. Jennifer, a thirty-five-year-old computer analyst from Santa Monica, California, says, "I have taken DMAE on numerous occasions over the last few months and have found that I get moody with high doses and start having arguments. Small doses are fine and help me become more alert and focused, but my problems come with amounts exceeding 350 mg of DMAE bitartrate."

The Author's Experience

Within two hours of taking 130 mg of actual DMAE, I notice a definite increase in alertness and slight mood and visual enhancement. I also get more motivated to work on projects and seem to work more efficiently. On higher doses I have experienced neck stiffness and anxiety.

Cautions and Side Effects

High doses can induce irritability, overstimulation, anxiety, headaches, and stiffness in the jaw, neck, and shoulder.

Recommendations

DMAE can be helpful in the elderly who have cognitive decline. This nutrient can also be taken by an adult of any age who needs to be more focused and alert.

Summary

Methyl donors are very interesting nutrients with a great deal of potential, particularly as antidepressants. Since our body's ability to methylate declines with age, it's possible that methyl donors someday may be found to have anti-aging benefits (Cooney 1993). These nutrients can also be taken on days when one needs to be more focused and alert.

In addition to their effects on the mind, methyl donors, along with B vitamins, can help lower homocysteine levels, thus reducing the risk for certain heart and neurological diseases.

ELEVEN

Keep Your Brain Young with Old and New Antioxidants

Just about everybody has heard the word **antioxidant.** Over the past few years, the benefits of antioxidants—such as vitamins C and E—have been touted in countless magazine and newspaper articles. Yet even with all this press, most people don't have a good understanding of the concept of oxidation and antioxidation. I recently asked a number of my patients if they really knew what the word *antioxidant* meant. Although the majority of these patients were taking antioxidants, only a few understood what they were or how they really worked.

UNDERSTANDING ANTIOXIDANTS

A common way used to describe "oxidation" is a piece of metal in the process of rusting; the process that occurs in the body is obviously different since we are made of living tissue: During the normal metabolism (or breakdown) of carbohydrates, fats, and proteins for energy production, certain molecules are generated that can damage the contents within cells. These destructive molecules often contain an unstable oxygen atom missing an electron. You may recall from high-school or college chemistry that atoms, such as hydrogen and oxygen, have a pair of electrons spinning around them. An atom with only one electron in its orbit is very unstable. Chemists call this atom a **free radical**. This free radical can then steal an electron from a neighboring molecule and hence cause that molecule to become damaged. The process of this damage is called **oxidation.** Cigarette smoke, fried foods, ozone, excessive sun exposure, car exhaust, certain drugs, radiation, toxins, and air pollution lead to free radical formation or direct oxidation.

The body has developed ways to counteract these oxidants, by producing antioxidants. An antioxidant is any chemical, natural or synthetic, that has the ability to neutralize oxidants, thus protecting our cells from being damaged. There's often a good balance between oxidation and antioxidation. A certain amount of oxidation in the body is necessary in order to fight infections or to do repair work within cells. However, when a shift occurs that leads to a preponderance of oxidation without adequate antioxidant support, the body undergoes what's called "oxidative stress." The body normally produces powerful natural antioxidants—such as superoxide dismutase, glutathione, and catalase—to help fight these oxidants. Many antioxidants are also consumed through the diet, particularly fresh fruits and vegetables.

When excessive oxidation occurs for prolonged periods, it can take a toll on the system. Changes occur in cells, including damage to fatty acids, inactivation of enzymes, deterioration of cell membranes, breakdown of proteins, and damage to the DNA. For instance, if oxidants damage DNA, the eventual consequence could be a higher likelihood of cancer. If the damage occurs in arteries that supply blood to the heart, it could lead to hardening of the arteries and a heart attack. All these changes lead to disease and premature aging.

Over the past few years, scientific evidence has slowly accumulated indicating that taking antioxidant supplements could potentially reduce the risk of certain illnesses and maintain brain health. There is, as of now, no proof that ingesting antioxidants prolongs the life span in humans, but enough evidence has been accumulated on the benefits of antioxidants that one should not casually dismiss their potential in improving quality of life and slowing the progression of certain chronic degenerative disorders.

But with the thousands of antioxidants available in our foodstuffs and the dozens available as supplements, which ones should you take, and in what dosages? This chapter will provide you with practical guidelines.

Brain Cells Can Get Oxidized

The cell membranes of neurons are made mostly of phospholipids, which contain fatty acids. Nerve fibers that travel from the brain to the spinal cord, and from the spinal cord to the rest of the body, are also insulated with a white-colored fatty substance called myelin. With time, these fats can become oxidized, interfering with proper nerve activity. The process of fats becoming oxidized is called "lipid peroxidation." The oxidation of fats contributes to brain aging and can accelerate degenerative disorders such as Alzheimer's disease. You may recall from Chapter 7 that the brain contains a great deal of polyunsaturated fatty acids, such as DHA and arachidonic acid, which are particularly susceptible to oxidation. As we age, many of these fatty acids in the brain become damaged due to oxidation and they lose some of their double bonds, thus becoming more saturated. Neurons in the brain become less efficient the more the fatty acids become saturated. Antioxidants can thus play a protective role in keeping the fatty acids in the brain healthy. After all, about 60 percent of the brain is made of fat.

Antioxidants and Memory

Although many antioxidant pills do not immediately influence cognition and memory, they very well could have a positive effect in the long run. Researchers at the University of Bern, in Switzerland, evaluated a total of 300 male and 130 female volunteers, over twenty-two years. In 1971, they measured blood levels of three antioxidants:

WHAT CAN ANTIOXIDANTS DO FOR YOU?

As a rule, you are not likely to notice any immediate cognitive benefits from taking the antioxidants discussed in this chapter. Therefore, do not expect any dramatic changes in mood, energy, alertness, or memory. Antioxidants can be compared to health insurance. You pay your monthly fee but don't often get the benefits until years later when you need a hospital bill paid. Antioxidants serve to protect your brain cells, proteins, and DNA from the gradual damage that occurs with the aging process. However, Chapter 12 will discuss other nutrients that have antioxidant benefits, such as CoQ10 and lipoic acid, which are mind energizers—they have immediate cognitive effects.

WHAT CONDITIONS DO ANTIOXIDANTS BENEFIT?

It's quite likely that, over the long run, antioxidants could slow the progression of age-related cognitive decline, Alzheimer's disease, Parkinson's disease, and perhaps other neurological disorders.

WHAT ARE SOME EXAMPLES OF OXIDANTS?

There are quite a number of damaging oxidants that we are exposed to on a daily basis. The most common are hydroxyl (OH), superoxide (O_2), hydrogen peroxide (H_2O_2), and ozone (O_3).

vitamin E, vitamin C, and beta-carotene. They also performed extensive memory testing. They found that higher levels of antioxidants, particularly vitamin C and beta-carotene, were associated with better performance in memory testing. The researchers state, "These results indicate the important role played by antioxidants in brain aging and may have implications for prevention of progressive cognitive impairments."

The researchers only tested blood levels of three antioxidants. It is quite likely that a number of other antioxidants play a role in helping us preserve memory and mental capacities in our later years. For instance, an eight-month study in rats showed administration of extracts from strawberries and spinach, either alone or with vitamin E, was able to slow damage to brain cells due to the aging process (Joseph 1998).

Dozens of antioxidant products are available over-the-counter. Please keep in mind that many foods, plants, herbal extracts, and other edible substances such as mushrooms, royal jelly, seaweed, and others, contain beneficial antioxidants and nutrients. In subsequent chapters I discuss a few nutrients and herbs, such as CoQ10, lipoic acid, and ginkgo, that also possess good antioxidant properties.

In this chapter I will briefly discuss some of the well-known antioxidants and also mention others that should be considered as part of a comprehensive antioxidant mind-preserving program.

VITAMIN C

Also known as ascorbic acid, vitamin C was isolated in 1928. This vitamin serves as an excellent antioxidant and could protect brain cells, including cells in the eye. The eye is highly susceptible to damage by sunlight, oxygen, various chemicals, and pollutants. Because of an aging Western-world population and a continued depletion of ozone, having adequate antioxidants in the eye is very important. But how much vitamin C is enough to protect our cells?

Ever since Nobel Prize winner Linus Pauling extolled the benefits of megadosing with vitamin C, the medical community has been debating the optimal dosage of this vitamin. Although many doctors stood firm for a long time, asserting that the RDA of 60 mg for this vitamin was adequate, more and more doctors are now realizing that higher doses can confer additional antioxidant benefits. However, the optimal daily intake of vitamin C has not yet been determined, nor is it likely to be determined soon. Nevertheless, we now suspect that excessive intake of vitamin C, expect perhaps in the therapy of a particular medical condition, may not be necessary.

A study published in the *American Journal of Clinical Nutrition* points that large doses of ingested vitamin C may be excreted without being utilized (Blanchard 1997). When the dosage of vitamin C given to a group of healthy men was increased from 200 mg a day to 2500 mg a day, blood levels increased only negligibly. James Blanchard, Ph.D., a professor of pharmacological sciences at the University of Arizona in Tucson, reports that the blood levels of vitamin C generally reflect the levels found in the rest of the body.

Recommendations

Most people should have adequate antioxidant protection with vitamin C at a dose of 100 to 500 mg per day. The majority of our intake of vitamin C should be obtained from fruits and vegetables, which additionally provide hundreds of beneficial carotenoids and flavonoids that often work synergistically with vitamin C.

Many people take more than one antioxidant on a daily basis. Since antioxidants help protect each other from being destroyed, the amount required for each one would be lessened when taken together.

VITAMIN E

Also known as tocopherol, vitamin E was isolated in the 1920s. There is general agreement that this fat-soluble vitamin can function as an excellent antioxidant, protecting cells from damage, and specifically protecting polyunsaturated fatty acids. Epidemiological studies indicate that older individuals with high levels of antioxidants in their bloodstream, including vitamin E, maintain a sharper memory (Perkins 1999).

Several types of natural vitamin-E compounds are available, including alpha-, beta-, gamma-, and delta-tocopherol. Alpha-tocopherol seems to be the most active, although we should not dismiss the importance of the others. It seems prudent to supplement with products that have mixed tocopherols as opposed to just alpha-tocopherol.

Recommendations

The average American diet contains between 10 and 22 international units of vitamin E. Additional intake is likely to be beneficial. Most healthy adults should do well with supplementing with 20 to 100 units a day. Very high dosages, such as 1000 units or more, can lead to an increase in bleeding risk, tiredness, and possibly impaired immune function.

CAROTENOIDS

These are a group of compounds that impart some of the orange color in vegetables and fruits. At least a few hundred of these carotenoids are found in our produce. Beta-carotene is the best known, but others are becoming more popular, including lycopene (found in tomatoes, watermelon, and much pink/red/orange-colored produce), lutein, zeazanthin, and others. Many carotenoids have antitumor, antibacterial, antiviral, anti-inflammatory, and antihistaminic actions. A diet rich in fruit and vegetables is likely to help prevent age-related mental decline.

Recommendations

Most healthy individuals do not need to take supplements of carotenoids since they can be easily found in produce. I recommend consuming a variety of foods and vegetables on a daily basis. There is a potential risk of causing an imbalance when supplementing with high doses of only one carotenoid, such as beta-carotene, at the expense of the others. It's possible, though, that someday we may discover that certain medical conditions may respond to supplementation with specific carotenoids.

FLAVONOIDS

Similar to the carotenoids, flavonoids are plant substances that have important antioxidant properties. Many of these also have antitumor, antibacterial, antiviral, anti-inflammatory, and antihistaminic actions. Some of the well-known flavonoids include quercetin, apigenin, rutin, and flavones. A certain type of flavonoids, called proanthrocyanidins, is found in extracts of pine bark and grape seeds. Polyphenols are another group of beneficial flavonoids. One such polyphenol, known as catechin, is found in green tea and other teas. You can find polyphenols in fruits, vegetables, herbs, wine, and certain legumes.

Recommendations

Flavonoid supplements are sold either individually, in combination with other flavonoids and carotenoids, or in combination with other nutrients. Most healthy individuals do not need to take supplements of flavonoids if they consume a healthy diet. I recommend your diet include a wide range of fruits (citrus, berries), grains, herbs, nuts, seeds, and vegetables (garlic, onions, broccoli).

It's possible we may someday determine that additional supplementation with specific flavonoids could potentially be beneficial in certain medical conditions.

GLUTATHIONE

This antioxidant, made from the combination of three amino acids, cysteine, glutamate, and glycine, forms part of the powerful natural antioxidant glutathione peroxidase (GP) which is found in our cells. GP plays a variety of roles in cells, including DNA synthesis and repair, metabolism of toxins and carcinogens, enhancement of the immune system, and prevention of fat oxidation. However, glutathione is predominantly known as an antioxidant protecting our cells from damage caused by the free-radical hydrogen peroxide. Glutathione also helps the other antioxidants in cells stay in their active form. Brain glutathione levels have been found to be lower in patients with Parkinson's disease.

Glutathione is found in foods, particularly fruits, vegetables, and meats. Cyanohydroxybutene, a chemical found in broccoli, cauliflower, brussels sprouts, and cabbage, is also thought to increase glutathione levels (Davis 1993). Although glutathione is available in pill form over-the-counter, its utilization by the body is questionable since we don't know if it can easily enter cells even after it is absorbed in the bloodstream.

Certain nutrients help raise tissue levels of glutathione, including NAC (see below), methyl donors, lipoic acid, and vitamin B_{12}. However, there appears to be a feedback inhibition in glutathione synthesis. This means that if glutathione levels are excessively increased with the help of nutrients, the body may decrease its natural production. The frequent use of acetaminophen (Tylenol) depletes glutathione levels.

Recommendations

Glutathione is sold in pills with doses ranging from 50 to 250 mg. Glutathione is a promising antioxidant. However, due to the inconsistencies in the medical literature on the ability of glutathione to enter tissues and cells when ingested orally, and the possibility of feedback inhibition, I can't confidently recommend supplementation with this nutrient until more information is published.

NAC (N-ACETYL-CYSTEINE)

I could have included NAC in Chapter 13, on amino acids and related compounds, since it is made from the amino acid cysteine. However, NAC is such a strong antioxidant that placing it in this chapter is more appropriate. NAC donates the amino acid cysteine to help form the antioxidant glutathione (Urban 1997).

An excellent review article in the April 1998 issue of *Alternative Medicine Reviews* summarizes the known effects of NAC (Kelly 1998). The author writes,

> N-acetyl-cysteine is an excellent source of sulfhydryl (SH) groups, and is converted in the body into metabolites capable of stimulating glutathione synthesis, promoting detoxification, and acting directly as a free-radical scavenger. Administration of NAC has historically been as a mucolytic [mucus dissolving] agent in a variety of respiratory illnesses; however, it appears to also have beneficial effects in conditions characterized by decreased glutathione or oxidative stress, such as HIV infection, cancer, heart disease, and cigarette smoking.

As a resident, I prescribed NAC intravenously to patients with liver damage due to acetaminophen (Tylenol) overdose. It protected the liver very well.

Cautions and Side Effects

Other than large doses causing nausea and vomiting, NAC is a safe nutrient. I experienced nausea for a few minutes within an hour of taking three 600 mg pills on an empty stomach. I did not notice any effect on mood or energy that day. One laboratory study indicates that while low dosages of NAC protect against oxidation, higher doses may have the opposite effect (Sprong 1998).

Recommendations

NAC is sold in dosages ranging from 250 to 600 mg. NAC can help form the powerful antioxidant glutathione, but you may recall that the formation of glutathione synthesis is under feedback control. Administration of NAC, with the resulting increase in glutathione levels, may cause a feedback inhibition in glutathione synthesis. Thus it is not clear whether regular use of NAC can actually increase overall glutathione levels in healthy individuals who have normal levels of glutathione. The use of NAC certainly should be considered as an additional supplement in protecting various cells from damage in the elderly and those with Parkinson's disease. If you are planning to use NAC along with other antioxidants, limit your daily dosage to 50 to 100 mg and don't take it all the time.

NAC could protect the livers of those who take acetaminophen on a regular basis.

SELENIUM

This mineral forms part of a very important enzyme normally present in our bodies, called glutathione peroxidase. The richest sources of selenium are organ meats and seafood, followed by meat, cereal products, and dairy.

The average intake of selenium in the American diet is 70 to 100 micrograms a day. Occasional supplementation with 20 to 100 micrograms of this mineral appears to be safe. Selenium in much higher amounts can act as an oxidant and thus is counterproductive (Spallholz 1997). As with most supplements, low-dose use seems to be a cautious approach.

Summary

Pick up any health magazine and you are likely to see ads promoting dozens of different antioxidants. Many of them have a scientific basis

ANTIOXIDANT DOSAGE GUIDELINES

Following is an antioxidant dosage recommendation for the average person who has no major medical problems. Please discuss with your health-care practitioner whether these doses are appropriate for your particular condition. Chapter 12 discusses additional nutrients—such as ALC, CoQ10, and lipoic acid—that are powerful antioxidants.

- Vitamin E—20 to 200 i.u. a day of the mixed tocopherols
- Vitamin C—100 to 500 mg a day
- Selenium—20 to 100 micrograms most days
- NAC—50 to 100 mg a few times a week
- Carotenoids and flavonoids are best obtained through fruits and vegetables

to support their antioxidant properties. However, you can't just take all of them. What should you do?

First, keep in mind that as of yet there is no definite proof that antioxidant supplements will keep your brain young. However, there is enough promising evidence to convince me to recommend the antioxidants mentioned in the sidebar.

Second, make sure you obtain the bulk of your antioxidants through fresh foods. Carotenoids and flavonoids can be easily obtained through fruits, vegetables, herbs, and whole foods. If you do wish to take additional supplements, I recommend a multioxidant pill that contains small amounts of many antioxidants, as opposed to large amounts of just one or two. You could even have two or three different products on your kitchen counter and alternate their use so you don't get the same antioxidants in the same dosages all the time. Remember that the body needs some oxidation in order to fight certain germs and possibly to fight some cancer cells.

TWELVE

Mind Energizers—Think Faster, Sharper, and Longer

Just like all the cells in the body, brain cells, or neurons, need energy. In most children and young adults, the brain is able to metabolize glucose and other sources of energy very well. However, as we get older, the energy production system in neurons doesn't seem to work as well. This malfunction could contribute to mental fatigue and the age-related decline in learning and memory.

This chapter will focus on three nutrients that are directly and actively involved in energy production: acetyl-L-carnitine (ALC), coenzyme Q10 (CoQ10), and lipoic acid. When used properly, these nutrients enhance mental function. CoQ10 is the best known of the three, and is used mostly in the treatment of cardiovascular conditions. ALC and lipoic acid have been available for several years and their popularity is gradually increasing. As an added benefit, all three of these mind-energizing nutrients also act as excellent antioxidants.

CoQ10 has become very popular over the past few years, as more people recognize the increase in energy it provides. Diane, a forty-six-year-old investment banker, says, "Ever since I started taking 30 mg of CoQ10 each morning, I seem to be peppy all day. I used to have a very mild case of chronic fatigue with slight fogginess of the mind. CoQ10 helps a lot, but sometimes I need 60 mg." ALC has its

WHAT CAN MIND ENERGIZERS DO FOR YOU?

The most obvious benefits noted from this group of nutrients are improvements in

- Alertness, arousal, and vigilance
- Mood, energy, and motivation
- Concentration and focus
- Verbal fluency
- Mild visual enhancement

WHAT CLINICAL CONDITIONS CAN MIND ENERGIZERS BENEFIT?

Limited research indicates that these nutrients can potentially be helpful in

- Depression
- Age-related cognitive decline
- Alzheimer's disease
- Parkinson's disease

share of fans, also. Renee, a fifty-five-year-old insurance agent, finds that this nutrient helps her stay focused all day. "I work with numbers all day," she says. "I take 250 mg of ALC on days when I want to be more alert and sharper. ALC improves my concentration and I actually feel smarter." Some diabetics currently take lipoic acid since this nutrient helps keep nerves healthier and stabilizes blood sugar levels. Few people are aware, though, that lipoic acid has cognitive benefits.

CARNITINE AND ALC (ACETYL-L-CARNITINE)

Carnitine is a naturally occurring substance found in most cells of the body, particularly the brain and neural tissues, muscles, and heart. Carnitine, whose structure is similar to choline, is widely available in animal foods and dairy products, whereas plants have very small amounts. Most non-vegetarians consume about 100 to 300 mg of carnitine a day, and the body is able to synthesize this nutrient if dietary intake is inadequate. When ingested as a pill, carnitine is not able to cross the blood-brain barrier as well as its activated form ALC can. ALC has significantly more noticeable cognitive effects than carnitine. This section, then, will focus on ALC.

How They Work

Carnitine and ALC play several important roles in the human body, particularly in energy metabolism. These nutrients shuttle acetyl groups and fatty acids into mitochondria for energy production. Without carnitine, fatty acids cannot easily enter into mitochondria. The acetyl group of ALC is used to form acetyl-CoA, the most important intermediary in the generation of energy from amino acids, fats, and carbohydrates. Therefore, ALC serves as an energy reservoir of acetyl groups and both ALC and carnitine help improve energy production. Those who take carnitine pills notice an increase in energy levels. The acetyl group of ALC is also used to make the important brain chemical acetylcholine. Some studies suggest that perhaps ALC can even act as a neurotransmitter itself.

In addition to producing energy, these two nutrients remove toxic accumulations of fatty acids from mitochondria, keeping these organelles healthy and functioning at their best (Carta 1993). Energy production in the mitochondria is not a perfect process, and toxic metabolites can often accumulate. Accumulation of these toxic metabolites and the resulting oxidative damage is likely to contribute to aging of cells (Shigenaga 1994). A waste substance called lipofuscin accumulates in cells as we age, and perhaps adequate ALC intake can help minimize this accumulation. A study in rats, providing them with ALC from their youth, showed this nutrient to decrease lipofuscin levels in their brain as they got older (Maccari 1990); therefore, it is theoretically possible that supplementation with carnitine or ALC can slow the aging process.

If the above benefits weren't enough, studies show that carnitine and ALC stabilize cell membranes, protect synapses, and protect neurons against damage from oxidation (Fariello, 1988).

Clinical Uses

ALC has been tested more often than carnitine in neurological conditions since, when ingested as a supplement, it can cross the blood-brain barrier very easily (Parnetti 1995). ALC can potentially be helpful in several groups of individuals, particularly those with Alzheimer's disease, age-related cognitive decline, and depression.

There are a few reasons why ALC may be helpful in Alzheimer's disease (AD). First, it helps form the important brain chemical acetylcholine, which is often deficient in AD. Second, ALC can clear toxic accumulations of fatty-acid metabolites from mitochondria, allowing for more efficient energy production. Third, it can potentially help regenerate cholinergic neurons. A study in rats has found that administration of ALC can induce the production of nerve-growth factor, a type of protein that helps regenerate neurons (Piovesan 1994). And last, some patients with AD may be deficient in the enzyme that converts carnitine to acetyl-L-carnitine (Kalaria 1992); therefore, providing ALC is an easy solution to this problem.

There have been several trials using ALC in the therapy of AD. The most extensive was a one-year-long double-blind, placebo-controlled study at the University of California San Diego in La Jolla, California (Thal 1996). The results were only slightly encouraging. Subjects with mild-to-moderate AD, aged 50-plus, were treated with 3 grams a day of ALC or placebo for twelve months. Four hundred thirty-one patients entered the study, and 83 percent completed one year of treatment. Overall, both ALC- and placebo-treated patients declined at the same rate on all cognitive measures during the trial. When the researchers examined the data more closely, they found that that those patients whose AD had started early (aged 65 years or younger at study entry) had a better response than those who were older than age 66 at the start of the study.

Here's a summary of additional research with ALC in Alzheimer's disease:

- A double-blind placebo-controlled study with seven AD patients was conducted over one year at the University of Pittsburgh in Pennsylvania (Pettegrew 1995). Compared to AD patients on placebo, acetyl-L-carnitine–treated patients showed significantly less deterioration.
- In a double-blind placebo-controlled clinical trial, researchers from the Mario Negri Institute for Pharmacological Research in Milan, Italy, studied the efficacy of a one-year treatment with 2 grams of ALC a day in 130 patients with AD (Spagnoli 1991). After one year, both the treated and placebo groups had worsened, but the treated group showed a slower rate of deterioration. The treated group showed better scores on logical intelligence, verbal critical abilities, and long-term verbal memory. Reported adverse events were relatively mild, and there was no significant difference between the treated and placebo groups either in incidence or severity of side effects.
- Investigators at Whittington Hospital in London, England, carried out a twenty-four week double-blind clinical trial comparing treatment with 1 gram ALC twice daily and a placebo in twenty patients with AD (Rai 1990). There was apparent improvement in the ALC group in tests on short-term memory. Laboratory tests revealed no signs of toxicity.
- ALC has also been tested in age-related cognitive decline. A 1990 study at the University of Parma showed that 2 grams a day of ALC improved memory, verbal fluency, and attention among thirty patients over the age of 65 suffering from mild mental im-

pairment (Passeri 1990). That same year, another Italian study on the effects of ALC on mildly impaired elderly was carried out on 236 subjects (Cipolli 1990). Each subject was treated for 150 days, and a battery of tests (investigating cognitive functioning, emotional state, and behavior) was administered. The results showed that treatment with ALC significantly increased the effectiveness of performance on all the measures of cognitive functioning and mood.

- ALC has even been tested in the therapy of depression and shown to be helpful in improving mood. Out of sixty subjects with low mood aged 60 to 80 years, half were given 3 grams a day of ALC while the other half received a placebo (Bella 1990). The results showed that treatment with ALC induced a significant reduction in the severity of depressive symptoms and also a significant improvement in quality of life. ALC is a promising nutrient, particularly for Alzheimer's disease and age-related cognitive decline.

Availability and Dosage

ALC is usually available at doses ranging between 100 and 500 mg. It is expensive, and cost may slow its popularity. Carnitine is available in a variety of doses ranging from 250 to 750 mg and is also sold as a powder.

An Expert's Opinion

Dr. Ascanio Polimeni, M.D., a neuroendocrinologist from Rome, has used ALC in his practice with hundreds of patients. He says, "I like ALC very much, especially when it's combined with other cognitive enhancers. My patients notice increased attentiveness and alertness, and improved mood. Older patients find ALC helps them think clearer and learn easier."

The Author's Experience

I notice the effects of ALC within two hours after taking a 500 mg pill; these effects are arousal and vigilance, along with mood improvement, and can last most of the day. The maximum dose I have taken is 1500 mg without experiencing a side effect. My patients report similar benefits.

Cautions and Side Effects

ALC and carnitine are very well tolerated. High doses of ALC, though, can induce nausea, restlessness, and agitation.

Recommendations

I believe ALC holds a great deal of promise and is currently underutilized, particularly in therapy for age-related cognitive decline. The role of ALC in Alzheimer's disease is still not fully understood but there is a good possibility that ALC could be helpful to some patients.

Carnitine could be a beneficial supplement for vegetarians at a dosage of 100 to 250 mg a day. Carnitine is also a useful supplement for treating fatigue.

COENZYME Q10

CoQ10, also known as ubiquinone or ubiquinol, is a naturally occurring nutrient in each cell. CoQ10 is found in foods, particularly in fish and meats. In addition to playing a significant role in the energy system of each of our cells, CoQ10 is an excellent antioxidant.

Studies of CoQ10 have mostly focused on its role in heart disease. However, CoQ10 has a role in brain function, too. Most of my patients who take CoQ10 notice that this nutrient provides energy and mental clarity.

How Does It Work?

Each cell in the body needs a source of energy to survive. Energy is produced from sugars, fats, and amino acids in mitochondria. CoQ10 exists naturally in our mitochondria and carries electrons involved in energy metabolism. CoQ10 is essential in the production of adenosine triphosphate (ATP), the basic energy molecule of each cell.

In the bloodstream, CoQ10 is mainly transported by lipoproteins such as LDL (low-density lipoproteins) and HDL (high-density lipoproteins). It is thought that CoQ10 is one of the first antioxidants to be depleted when LDL is subjected to oxidation. Hence, CoQ10 is an extremely important nutrient that prevents the oxidation of lipoproteins, thus protecting arteries from forming plaques and getting damaged.

CoQ10 and the Brain

Studies evaluating the role of this nutrient in cognitive disorders are limited. Here are summaries of two important ones that have been published over the past few years.

- Parkinson's disease: Levels of coenzyme Q10 are lower in mitochondria from Parkinsonian patients than in mitochondria from age- and sex-matched controls (Shults 1997). However, limited clinical trials with this nutrient in the therapy of PD have not shown noticeable benefits. A three-month trial was performed to evaluate the efficacy of 200 mg of CoQ10 daily in ten patients with PD. There was no significant effect on the clinical ratings (Stijks 1997). A year later, another study again did not show any dramatic improvements when 200 mg of CoQ10 was administered two, three, or four times per day for one month in fifteen subjects with Parkinson's disease (Shults 1998).
- Juvenile neuronal ceroid lipofuscinosis (JNCL) is an inherited, progressive neurodegenerative disease. In this study the levels of the antioxidants CoQ10 and vitamin E were measured in blood samples of twenty-nine JNCL patients and compared to forty-eight healthy controls (Westermarck 1997). A significant reduction of the CoQ10 level was observed in JNCL patients when compared to control subjects. The level of vitamin E was also markedly reduced in JNCL patients when compared to controls.

> The low levels of CoQ10 and vitamin E in JNCL patients may indicate an impaired antioxidant protection in this disease.

Availability and Dosage

CoQ10 is sold in 10 to 100 mg capsules, and is also added to some multivitamin tablets.

The Author's Experience

The effect from 30 mg of CoQ10 is mild, mostly consisting of a slightly higher energy level. The effects become more noticeable with 60 mg. I have taken up to 120 mg in the morning. On this dose, I notice an increase in energy as the day goes on, with an urge to take a long walk or be otherwise physically active. There is a slight mood elevation with enhanced focus, motivation, and productivity, along with the desire to talk to people. The 120-mg dose, though, is too much, since I feel too energetic and alert even in late evening when I want to slow down and get ready for sleep.

Cautions and Side Effects

High dosages can induce restlessness and insomnia. *Since it has a chemical structure similar to vitamin K, patients taking blood thinners such as coumadin should probably avoid CoQ10, or keep their dosages low* (Landbo 1998).

Recommendations

CoQ10 will likely be found to play a positive role in certain cognitive or neurodegenerative disorders, but more studies are needed. The results of short-term studies in Parkinson's disease have not been encouraging, although it is possible that the long-term use of CoQ10 in small doses may protect brain cells from oxidative damage. In the meantime, it would seem appropriate to supplement with this nutrient as part of a long-term health regimen. A daily dose of 10 to 30 mg seems to be a reasonable option for many individuals.

LIPOIC ACID

Lipoic acid (LA) is a natural coenzyme important in the regulation of carbohydrate metabolism. Lipoic acid is also slowly becoming recognized as having some unique and powerful antioxidant abilities. I could have included LA in the chapter on antioxidants but chose to place it in this chapter since, unlike other antioxidants such as vitamins E and C, LA is more clearly involved in energy production, and provides noticeable cognitive effects. Over the past few years this nutrient has been tested in the treatment and prevention of a broad range of diseases, including diabetes and diabetic neuropathy.

LA is often mentioned in the medical literature as alpha-lipoic acid or "thiotic acid." Although LA is found in small amounts in foods (such as meats and spinach), full evaluations of LA in food contents have not been done as well as they have been for other nutrients.

LA has some particularly useful antioxidant properties. It can help preserve the function of vitamins C and E, and increase the levels of glutathione, a very important antioxidant normally found in our cells (Busse 1992). Glutathione is an important natural antioxidant in the brain, particularly for patients with Parkinson's disease. Dr. Lester Packer and colleagues from the University of California at Berkeley have done extensive studies with LA (Packer 1997). They say,

> The metabolic antioxidant alpha-lipoate is absorbed from the diet and crosses the blood-brain barrier. Alpha-lipoate offers antioxidant protection to both intracellular [within a cell] and extracellular [outside a cell] environments. This potent antioxidant can regenerate other antioxidants like vitamin C and vitamin E, and raises intracellular glutathione levels. Thus, it would seem an ideal substance in the treatment of oxidative brain and neural disorders involving free-radical processes.

Dr. Packer tells me that research on lipoic acid and the brain thus far has been done only with animals and no studies are available regarding the cognitive role lipoic acid plays in humans.

Role in Neural Disorders and Memory

Nerves constantly use a lot of energy and thus are vulnerable to oxidative stress. In order to produce energy, nerve cells have a large number of mitochondria. Energy production produces free radicals, which can damage the DNA within cells. It's possible that an inadequate antioxidant defense system can lead to degenerative disorders of the nervous system.

Studies with LA and cognition are limited. When aging mice were given LA for fifteen days, they performed slightly better in a memory test than their younger counterparts given LA (Stoll 1993), and the number of NMDA receptors in brain cells improved (NMDA, which stands for N-methyl-D-aspartate, is a type of receptor involved with memory). Treatment with LA did not improve memory in young mice. LA has been used therapeutically in the therapy of diabetic neuropathy with moderate success.

Availability and Dosage

LA is sold in dosages of 50 and 100 mg but most do not need doses this high. You can open a capsule and take a small portion, such as 5 to 20 mg. You will also find lipoic acid added to certain multioxidant products in combinations with vitamins E, C, and CoQ10.

The Author's Experience

Unlike most antioxidants such as vitamins C, E, and selenium, there is actually a noticeable effect from taking LA. I've observed a sense of relaxed well-being and slightly enhanced visual acuity. Higher dosages, such as 40 mg or more, even when taken in the morning, cause me to have insomnia.

Cautions and Side Effects

There are no indications that low doses of LA, such as 5 to 20 mg, have side effects. Higher doses could cause nausea or stomach upset, along with overstimulation, fatigue, and insomnia. High doses could also potentially lower blood sugar. This is often beneficial to patients who have diabetes, but it requires close monitoring of blood-sugar levels.

Recommendations

Until long-term studies with LA are published on humans, I do not recommend that you take more than 20 mg a day unless you're being treated for a particular condition under medical supervision. Since LA helps restore antioxidants, take less vitamins C and E and other antioxidants when you take them along with LA.

Summary

There are a number of supplements available that influence energy production in brain cells. The research with all of these nutrients is still very early and it's difficult to give precise dosage recommendations or combinations that would apply to everyone.

I am very confident that with time more doctors will realize the enormous benefit some of these mind energizers can provide to individuals with a number of neurological and psychological conditions. I believe that the medical profession is currently underutilizing CoQ10, ALC, and lipoic acid.

Since carnitine and CoQ10 are mostly found in meat, fish, and chicken, I recommend vegetarians supplement with 100 to 250 mg of carnitine and 10 to 20 mg of CoQ10 on a regular basis.

THIRTEEN

Amino Acids: Building Blocks for Brain Chemicals

Sharon is a thirty-four-year-old housewife who can't get going in the morning without a caffeine boost. It takes her a couple of hours before she feels alert and ready to function. Sharon asked me whether there were any nutrients that would provide the type of "wake-up" alertness equivalent to a cup of coffee. I recommended she try a small dose of an amino acid called tyrosine, which she found worked very well. She now takes this amino acid once or so a week in the morning on an empty stomach. It makes her more focused and alert, often within an hour.

Mindy is a forty-five-year-old health-food-store manager who takes 5-HTP a few times a month near bedtime. "Whenever I'm very tense and know that I'm going to have trouble sleeping, I take 50 mg of 5-HTP about an hour before bed on an empty stomach. 5-HTP helps me get a restful sleep," she says.

There are a number of amino acids and related nutrients that are sold over-the-counter. Some of these include tyrosine, phenylalanine, 5-HTP, creatine, GABA, pyroglutamic acid, taurine, glutamine, and arginine. Sharon and Mindy are two individuals who have found that the occasional use of amino acids helps improve the quality of their lives. This chapter will discuss the appropriate use of tyrosine, 5-HTP, and phenylalanine. I have chosen to focus on these three amino acids because there is ample research, and a great deal of clinical experience, supporting their use. The other amino acids and related nutrients mentioned above are recommended for different purposes. For instance, creatine is a nutrient that increases muscle mass but has no cognitive effects. GABA, short for gamma-aminobutyric acid, is a brain chemical involved in relaxation but you won't notice much if you take a GABA pill. This is because GABA cannot easily cross the blood-brain barrier. Pyroglutamic acid does increase alertness and focus, but there is very little research published with this nutrient. Taurine, glutamine, and arginine have minimal cognitive effects.

What Is an Amino Acid?

The foods we eat contain proteins, fats, and carbohydrates. Proteins are made from many amino acids assembled into long chains. There are about twenty different types of amino acids that make up proteins. An amino acid is basically a molecule that combines an amino group (NH3) and a carboxyl group (COOH) attached to a side chain. The side chain gives each of the twenty different amino acids its unique property. Eight of the twenty amino acids are essential, that is, the body cannot manufacture them and hence they have to be ingested through foods. These essential amino acids include isoleucine, lysine, leucine, methionine, phenylalanine, threonine, tryptophan, and valine. The nonessential amino acids are alanine, arginine, asparagine, aspartate, cysteine, glutamate, glutamine, glycine, histidine, proline, serine, and tyrosine. In addition to the twenty common amino acids used to make proteins, there are others, such as taurine and pyroglutamate, that are not incorporated into proteins.

PHENYLALANINE AND TYROSINE

Phenylalanine is an essential amino acid, but tyrosine isn't since it can be made from phenylalanine. These two amino acids are converted

WHAT CAN AMINO ACIDS DO FOR YOU?

Tyrosine and phenylalanine are converted into the brain chemicals dopamine and norepinephrine. They lead to alertness, appetite control, and slight mood elevation. 5-HTP is converted into serotonin and induces relaxation, controls appetite, helps with sleep, and elevates mood.

WHAT CLINICAL CONDITIONS CAN AMINO ACIDS BENEFIT?

All three of these amino acids are useful in treating depression and obesity. 5-HTP can also be used in anxiety disorders and insomnia.

into dopamine and norepinephrine (see Figure 13.1). Supplementation with these amino acids leads to alertness, arousal, and more energy.

Phenylalanine and tyrosine are sometimes prescribed as antidepressants, usually in combination with other nutrients and herbs that have mood-elevating properties. Some doctors also recommend these amino acids for appetite control. Phenylalanine may trigger the release of an appetite-suppressing hormone in the gut called cholecystokinin. Most individuals who take either of these amino acids notice improved alertness, arousal, and mood, and a slight loss in appetite. I have a few patients who occasionally take a small amount of these nutrients—such as 50 to 250 mg—in the morning as a substitute for caffeine.

Availability and Dosage

Phenylalanine and tyrosine are sold in dosages ranging from 100 to 500 mg. Tyrosine is also sold in its acetylated form as acetyl-tyrosine. No human research has been published regarding the mental effects of acetyl-tyrosine compared to plain tyrosine.

Figure 13.1—Conversion of Phenylalanine and Tyrosine to Dopamine and Norepinephrine

Phenylalanine

▼ **(NADH)**

Tyrosine

▼ **Vitamin C**

L-Dopa

▼ **Vitamin B_6**

Dopamine

▼ **Vitamin C**

Norepinephrine

▼ **SAMe and methyl donors**

Epinephrine

Always start with a low dose, such as 50 to 100 mg, in order to avoid side effects. If you can only find the 500 mg pills, you may have to open a capsule and take a portion. The effects of tyrosine and phenylalanine are more noticeable when taken on an empty stomach.

Be careful when you are adding either of these two amino acids to a regimen that includes other stimulants since the effects can be cumulative. Some of the nutrients that can act as stimulants include DMAE, CDP-choline, pantothenic acid, methyl donors, ALC, CoQ10, DHEA, pregnenolone, St. John's wort, and ginseng.

The Author's Experience

I notice the effects from these amino acids with a dose as low as 100 mg when taken on an empty stomach in the morning. In addition to enhanced alertness, arousal, focus, and motivation, there is some appetite suppression and slight mood improvement. However, high doses make me anxious and restless. I have occasionally experienced brief episodes of heart palpitations when my dosage exceeded 750 mg.

I have taken acetyl-tyrosine twice, at a dose of 200 mg. The effects lasted most of the day and were similar to a higher dose of tyrosine.

Cautions and Side Effects

In high doses, these amino acids cause anxiety, restlessness, irritability, and insomnia. They also raise blood pressure, increase heart rate, and may even cause heart irregularities in susceptible individuals. Those who have a defect in the enzyme phenylalanine hydroxylase cannot easily metabolize phenylalanine to tyrosine, and develop a condition known as phenylketonuria. Obviously, these individuals should avoid phenylalanine.

Avoid these two amino acids if you are currently taking antidepressant drugs such as monoamine oxidase inhibitors (MAOs). Caution is also advised when they are used with serotonin reuptake inhibitors such as Prozac. Both phenylalanine and tyrosine can have a stimulant effect when combined with energizing nutrients and drugs. Because tyrosine is a precursor to thyroid hormones, individuals with thyroid problems should consult their physician before use.

Recommendations

Phenylalanine and tyrosine are useful in the therapy of depression and appetite control, especially when combined with other nutrients. I do not recommend their use for older individuals or for those who have high blood pressure, cardiovascular disease, or a propensity for heart palpitations.

Figure 13.2—Conversion of Tryptophan into 5-HTP, Serotonin, and Melatonin

Tryptophan

▼

5-Hydroxytryptophan (5-HTP)

▼ **Vitamin B_6**

Serotonin

▼

N-acetyl-serotonin

▼ **SAMe (and other methyl donors?)**

Melatonin

5-HTP (5-HYDROXYTRYPTOPHAN)

During the 1980s, consumers were using the amino acid tryptophan for sleep and as an antidepressant. Tryptophan was available up until 1989 when the FDA prohibited its over-the-counter sale, because a tryptophan manufacturer in Japan shipped a contaminated batch to the U.S. that caused a serious illness called eosinophilia myalgia syndrome. Tryptophan is now available only by prescription through compounding pharmacies. No further tryptophan contamination has been reported.

Since 1995, though, 5-HTP, the immediate precursor to serotonin, has been available without a prescription. Figure 13.2 shows that tryptophan converts into 5-HTP, which then readily converts into serotonin. Once serotonin is made, the pineal gland is able to convert it at night into melatonin, the sleep-inducing hormone.

The 5-HTP currently sold over-the-counter is extracted from griffonia seeds, which come from an African shrubtree grown in Ghana and the Ivory Coast. There are several European pharmaceutical companies that extract 5-HTP from these seeds.

Over the past three decades, scientists have tested 5-HTP for the following conditions:

- Anxiety disorders—Due to its conversion into serotonin, 5-HTP, when used occasionally, can induce relaxation and relieve anxiety.
- Depression—Most individuals find a slight mood elevation after using 5-HTP for a few days. Until more research is available, the regular use of 5-HTP as an antidepressant should be limited to a few weeks.
- Insomnia—The occasional use of 5-HTP in a dosage of 25 to 50 mg, about an hour before bed on an empty stomach, can help induce and maintain sleep.
- Obesity—5-HTP acts as a good appetite suppressant and can, in combination with lifestyle and dietary changes, help in weight reduction. Although 5-HTP can help one lose weight, this nutrient should only be used temporarily (a few weeks at most) until lifestyle habits are incorporated.

Availability and Dosage

5-HTP is sold in 25 to 100 mg capsules. Most people notice the effects from 10 to 50 mg when taken on an empty stomach.

The Author's Experience

I have tried 5-HTP on numerous occasions and have noticed that it can induce relaxation, improve mood, reduce hunger, and is effective for insomnia when used an hour or so before bed on an empty stomach. Tolerance to 5-HTP seems to develop rather quickly when it's taken frequently. The daytime side effects I've noticed on a dose greater than 50 mg include nausea and sluggishness. I've also had vivid dreams, including nightmares, on an evening dose of 100 mg.

Cautions and Side Effects

Due to limited available research on this nutrient, caution is advised. 5-HTP should only be used for a brief period, such as a few weeks. After a break of a month or two, 5-HTP can be restarted again.

Do not take a dose exceeding 25 mg during the day if you expect to drive a car or operate heavy machinery since 5-HTP can make some people sleepy. High doses, greater than 100 mg, can induce nausea. A high dose at night can cause vivid dreams and nightmares. The risk for side effects increases with the dose.

Recommendations

5-HTP can be helpful, most likely in combination with other nutrients, in treating obesity, anxiety, insomnia, and depression. *Until more studies are available, I recommend not using 5-HTP more than four days a week, and continuously no longer than a few weeks without taking breaks.* It takes time to learn how to use 5-HTP well.

Summary

Amino acids and their derivatives have very important functions in the brain and body. When used appropriately, they can offer a number of benefits in the therapy of mood disorders, anxiety, and appetite control. The medical profession has not taken full advantage of their potential uses.

FOURTEEN

Brain Hormones—Potent Memory and Sex Boosters

For many years we've heard about estrogen-replacement therapy and how it's supposed to fight osteoporosis, improve heart function, and help with some of the changes in mood that occur in menopause. We've also heard that testosterone replacement can improve sexual function and feelings of well-being. It is becoming apparent that steroid hormones, which include estrogen, testosterone, DHEA, progesterone, and pregnenolone, not only play important roles in the body, but also have a significant influence on brain function. These hormones are made mostly in the adrenal glands, ovaries, and testicles. However, many people don't realize that they are also made in the brain and have important effects on mental function. Since these hormones are made in neural tissue, scientists have proposed the name *neurohormones* to recognize and emphasize the importance of these hormones in the nervous system.

How hormones affect learning, memory, mood, and libido is still being investigated, but researchers have discovered that hormones can influence the activity of brain chemicals, the structure of receptors and synapses, the release of other hormones, DNA formation within brain cells, and communication within nerve cells (Rupprecht 1999). These are all very important influences.

WHAT CAN BRAIN HORMONES DO FOR YOU?

DHEA and pregnenolone are very powerful. If used appropriately, you can expect improvements in learning and memory, sex drive and sexual enjoyment, mood and energy, speed of thinking, verbal fluency, concentration and focus, creativity, vision, hearing, awareness, and sensory perception. Melatonin helps improve sleep.

WHAT CLINICAL CONDITIONS CAN BRAIN HORMONES BENEFIT?

Hormones have a broad range of effects, and if used properly, can have an influence in age-related cognitive decline, depression, and perhaps Alzheimer's disease. They also help improve libido in those who have lost interest in sex.

When we're young, particularly in our teens, we have adequate production of these hormones, but levels decline with age. Hormone supplements are generally reserved for those in their mid-forties and older. This chapter will focus on three hormones available over-the-counter: DHEA, pregnenolone, and melatonin.

CHOLESTEROL: THE SOURCE OF STEROID HORMONES

Cholesterol is one of the components of brain-cell membranes, and is also the precursor from which all steroid hormones are formed, not only in the adrenal glands, ovaries, and testicles, but also in the brain. As you can see from Figure 14.1, pregnenolone, DHEA, progesterone, estrogen, and testosterone are all formed from cholesterol.

Several studies over the past few years have indicated that drastically lowering cholesterol levels with drugs may lead to cognitive

Figure 14.1—The Making of Steroid Hormones from Cholesterol

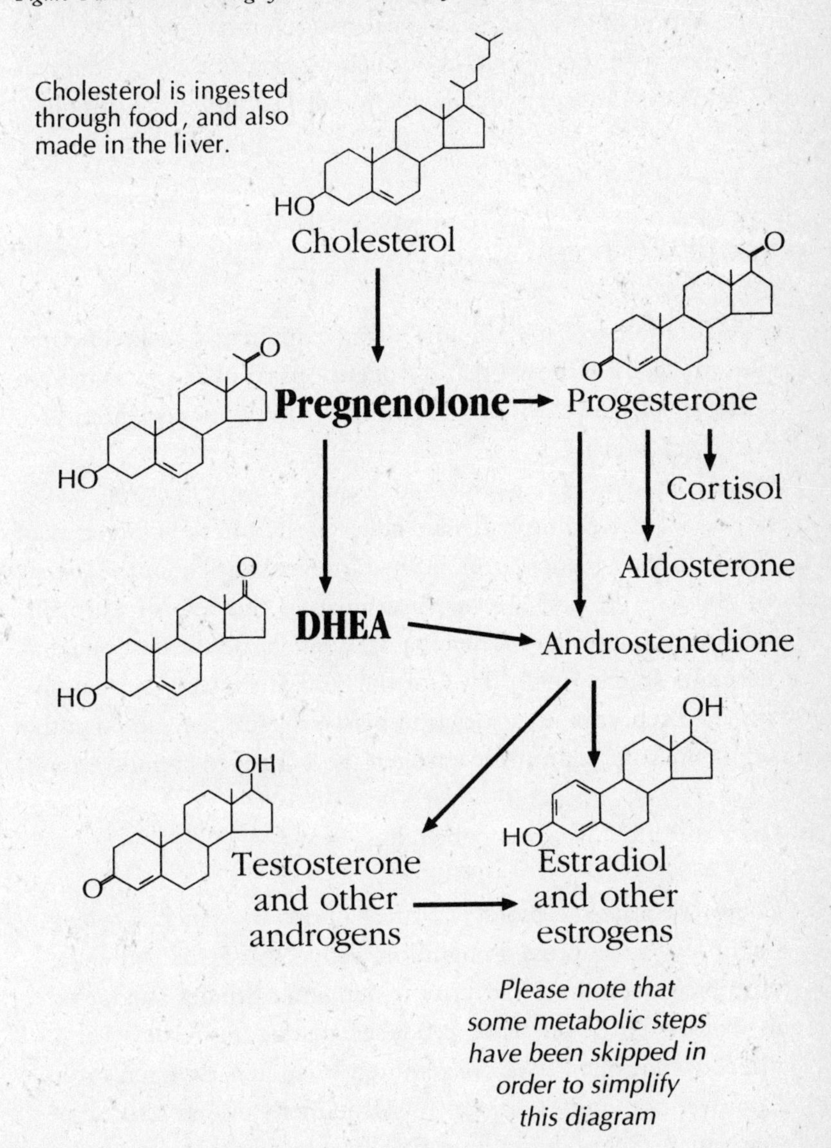

Please note that some metabolic steps have been skipped in order to simplify this diagram

decline, depression, and increased rates of suicide, homicide, and accidents. Although the reasons for this are not completely clear, could interference with the production of neurosteroids be one of the reasons? Additional research will likely provide the answers to this question.

ESTROGEN AND THE BRAIN

Scientists are still determining how estrogen influences brain function. Studies in rats have shown that estrogens can regulate the formation of synapses, alter levels of brain chemicals, and influence various receptors (McEwen 1997).

As we all know, there is a marked decline in levels of estrogen after menopause. Dr. Kristine Yaffe and colleagues, from the University of California in San Francisco, published a review article in the *Journal of the American Medical Association* evaluating the role of estrogen-replacement therapy in postmenopausal women and its effect on mental function (Yaffe 1998). Two of the studies showed inconclusive results, two reported no association between estrogen and cognitive function, and one found that estrogen use improved cognitive function.

Dr. Yaffe and colleagues conclude,

> There are plausible biological mechanisms by which estrogen might lead to improved cognition, reduced risk for dementia, or improvement in the severity of dementia. Studies conducted in women, however, have produced conflicting results. Large placebo-controlled trials are required to address estrogen's role in prevention and treatment of Alzheimer's disease and other dementias. Given the known risks of estrogen therapy, we do not recommend estrogen for the prevention or treatment of Alzheimer's disease or other dementias until adequate trials have been conducted.

Estrogens, unlike DHEA and pregnenolone, are available only through a doctor's prescription. Recently, plant estrogens, such as those found in soybeans or certain herbs, have become more popular. Further studies will determine whether a high intake of plant estrogens can reduce the required dosages of estrogen. In the meantime, the benefits and risks of estrogen replacement are still a matter of debate within the medical community, but most agree that a small dose of estrogen replacement may benefit some women.

Beyond Estrogen

During routine hormone-replacement therapy to postmenopausal women, doctors prescribe mainly estrogen (and sometimes progesterone or a synthetic progestin). Research is slowly accumulating, though, that suggests replacing small amounts of other hormones could potentially be helpful—not only for women, but men, too.

But not all the hormones in our bodies decline with age. Cortisol, made by the adrenal glands, and insulin, made by the pancreas, stay relatively the same, or even increase. Thyroid hormone levels vary. Pregnenolone, DHEA, growth hormone, progesterone, estrogens, and testosterone decrease with age.

The decline in the production of hormones due either to aging, or as a consequence of illness or chronic stress, can have a negative impact on a number of body tissues. All these hormones have the ability to enter most cells of the body, go to the DNA, induce the formations of a variety of enzymes and proteins, and significantly influence the function of cells and tissues.

Do Middle-Aged and Older Women Need Male Hormones?

Over the past two or more decades, women have been given estrogen not only for hot flashes, but also as hormone-replacement therapy to counteract osteoporosis and decrease the incidence of heart disease and stroke. Recently some doctors have started using testosterone replacement in both men and women. There's a 30 to 50 percent decline in testosterone levels in women between the ages of 20 and

50 (Zumoff, 1995). Furthermore, the ovaries after menopause stop making testosterone and estrogens. The decline in testosterone levels often leads to impaired sexual function, decreased feelings of well-being, loss of energy, and thinning of bones; therefore, some women are prescribed both estrogen and testosterone supplements.

The option of testosterone replacement should be given to post-menopausal women who suffer persistent loss of a sense of well-being, fatigue, and most commonly, loss of libido, despite adequate estrogen replacement and after exclusion of other possible underlying medical conditions. However, the benefits and risks of testosterone replacement are currently not fully known. Side effects of excessive testosterone use include acne and hair loss.

As you saw in from Figure 14.1, DHEA is eventually converted into both testosterone and estrogen. Therefore, DHEA is potentially an alternative means of replacing testosterone in older women.

DHEA: THE PARENT OF ESTROGEN AND TESTOSTERONE

Judy, a fifty-two-year-old travel agent married for twenty-four years, was having problems with her marriage. She told me,

> A few years ago, I noticed a distance develop between me and my husband. I just didn't have the urge to be intimate; and obviously, this hurt our closeness. The problem was getting worse and I really thought we were going to break up. I heard about DHEA, that it had the ability to improve sex drive. I started on 5 mg a day, and within a week, I couldn't keep my hands off my husband. He loved it. Now I only take the DHEA two or three times a week, and that seems to be sufficient.

What Benefits Does DHEA Provide?

DHEA is short for dehydroepiandrosterone, a hormone made mostly by the adrenal glands, located above the kidneys, but also made in the testicles, ovaries, and brain. After production in the adrenal glands, DHEA travels in the bloodstream and enters tissues and cells where it is converted to testosterone and estrogens.

Most long-term studies indicate that this hormone is able to provide a sense of well-being and improve energy levels in the majority of the users (Yen 1995, Labrie 1997). My clinical experience is consistent with the research findings. Owen Wolkowitz, M.D., from the Department of Psychiatry at the University of San Francisco, has been researching the role of DHEA as an antidepressant in middle-aged and older individuals. He tells me, "Our research has shown that DHEA supplementation improves mood."

In a double-blind German study published in the *New England Journal of Medicine*, twenty-four women with adrenal deficiency were given 50 mg of DHEA daily for four months (Wiebke 1999); adrenal insufficiency leads to a deficiency of dehydroepiandrosterone. DHEA supplements helped improve feelings of well-being, and increased the frequency of sexual thoughts and sexual interest.

DHEA is converted in the body into testosterone and it is well known that testosterone increases sexual drive. In my clinical experience, at least a third of men and women who take DHEA report an increase in sex drive.

Availability and Dosage

DHEA is sold as pills, cream, sublingual tablets, and time-release pills. Capsules and pills are sold in doses of 5 mg upward to 100 mg. Side effects (see below) are common on doses greater than 10 mg. I hope more vitamin companies provide the 5 mg pills and stop selling the higher doses.

Androstenedione is also available over-the-counter. I call it the "son of DHEA" since it is made from DHEA and has similar functions. Studies with androstenedione are much more limited that those with DHEA and at this point it is difficult to predict which of the two is a better choice in hormone replacement.

A new form of DHEA, called 7-keto DHEA, was introduced in

1998. The companies promoting this product claim that it does not convert to testosterone and estrogen and hence does not have androgenic and estrogenic side effects. On the other hand, they claim that 7-keto DHEA provides similar, or better, benefits than DHEA. If 7-keto DHEA does not convert into testosterone, as is claimed, then it is unlikely to have a significant effect on libido. No significant human trials have been published with 7-keto DHEA in peer-reviewed journals; therefore, it is premature to make any definitive claims regarding the use of 7-keto DHEA.

Cautions and Side Effects

- Although DHEA can clearly improve mental function, users should be cautious. The influence of long-term DHEA supplementation on human tumor initiation, promotion, or inhibition is not known at this time. DHEA could increase the risk for benign prostatic enlargement. High doses, generally more than 20 mg, may lead to heart palpitations in those prone to arrhythmias (Sahelian 1998). In order to reduce the risk for heart palpitations, make sure you have an adequate intake of fish oils and magnesium. If your medical condition requires that you take high doses of DHEA, have your doctor prescribe you a few pills of a beta-blocker such as propranolol to carry with you. Take 40 to 60 mg of propranol if you suddenly develop a palpitation.
- Side effects can readily occur with the misuse of DHEA. These side effects are clearly dose-dependent, and generally begin at about 5 mg. Individuals prone to acne can get pimples on a dose as low as 2 mg. Women can experience hair growth in unwanted places such as the face and chin. DHEA could lead to accelerated scalp-hair loss due to this hormone's conversion into dihydrotestosterone (DHT), the hormone associated with hair loss. If you experience hair loss, stop the DHEA. Ask your doctor whether temporary therapy with finasteride (available in 5 mg doses as Proscar or a 1 mg dose as Propecia) might be appropriate. Finas-

teride blocks the conversion of testosterone to DHT and can regrow hair.

- Anecdotal information indicates that high dosages of DHEA can lead to menstrual irregularities, overstimulation, occasional nervousness, irritability, aggressiveness, headaches, and mood changes. Evaluation and supervision by a health-care provider is strongly advised when supplementing with hormones.

Recommendations

There is little doubt that many individuals, especially those whose adrenal glands produce low levels of DHEA, notice an improvement in mood and sex drive when supplementing with this hormone. Some even report an improvement in energy, memory, and thinking abilities. However, due its potential androgenic side effects such as hair loss, and unknown long-term effects, I urge individuals to use the least amount possible and to take breaks from use, which I call "hormone holidays." See the end of the chapter for dosage guidelines.

PREGNENOLONE: THE GRANDMOTHER OF ALL STEROID HORMONES

Bill, a sixty-eight-year-old engineer from Park City, Utah, says, "I find pregnenolone to be a powerful memory booster. Ever since I started taking 5 mg three times a week, I remember phone numbers and names much easier."

Most users of pregnenolone (Preg), find this hormone to help with learning and memory, mood and energy, speed of thinking, verbal fluency, concentration and focus, creativity, vision, hearing, awareness, and sensory perception. Some even report an enhancement in sex drive and sexual enjoyment.

Preg is primarily made in the adrenal glands from cholesterol, but it can also be made in other tissues, including the brain. I call Preg the "grandmother of all the steroid hormones" since the body uses it to convert into DHEA, progesterone, and other steroid hormones (see Figure 14.1). Human research with Preg is very limited but several rodent studies have shown it to be a powerful memory enhancer (Flood 1995).

Availability and Dosage

Pills and sublingual tablets are sold in doses starting at 5 mg upward to 50 mg. Maximum regular, daily dosage should not exceed 5 mg. I recommend that you take hormone holidays similar to DHEA. Both Preg and DHEA have overlapping functions; therefore, if you plan to add Preg to your DHEA regimen, you need to reduce your dosage of DHEA. Preg is best taken in the morning, or no later than noon.

I'm often asked, if Preg, "the grandmother of all steroid hormones" can be converted into DHEA, progesterone, and the other steroid hormones, why not use it exclusively, and let the body convert it into the specific steroid hormones it requires?

Young people have the ability to easily convert Preg into all the other steroid hormones. As we age, the enzymes that convert Preg to DHEA, and Preg to progesterone, may not work as well. Nor would the enzymes that convert DHEA into androgens and estrogens be as effective. Therefore, in older individuals, giving Preg alone may not be enough.

Users' Experiences

I have recommended pregnenolone to dozens of patients. The majority reports that this hormone enhances alertness and arousal, and has a profound effect on memory and awareness. At least a third notice an enhancement in visual perception. A few find an increase in sexual enjoyment, but the sexual effects are not as consistent as that of DHEA.

Many older patients report that pregnenolone helps them recall phone numbers and names. One seventy-two-year-old patient says, "Before I started pregnenolone, I often found myself starting a sentence and forgetting what I was saying. Pregnenolone has been amazing. I never have problems with finishing sentences anymore. Both my short-term and long-term memory seem to be vastly improved."

The Author's Experience

I have taken pregnenolone on numerous occasions at doses ranging from 2 to 60 mg. Pregnenolone improves my visual and auditory perception along with providing a sense of well-being. I have also experienced side effects of headaches, acne, insomnia, irritability, and heart palpitations on doses greater than 20 mg. I use Preg only two or three times a month, on days when I need to be more alert and focused. Sometimes I take Preg if I wish to improve my visual appreciation, such as when I plan to visit an art gallery or an antique show. For instance, in March of 1999 I visited a Van Gogh exhibit at the Los Angeles County Museum of Art. That morning I had taken 10 mg of Preg along with ten capsules of fish oils. This combination certainly made my visit to the exhibit much more enjoyable.

Cautions and Side Effects

High doses can lead to androgenic side effects similar to those of DHEA, including acne and accelerated hair loss. Irritability, aggressiveness, insomnia, anxiety, headaches, and menstrual irregularities are also frequently reported in doses greater than 10 mg. *Heart palpitations can occur in doses greater than 20 mg, or even at 5 mg in individuals prone to irregular rhythms.*

- In order to reduce the risk for heart palpitations, make sure you have an adequate intake of fish oils and magnesium. If your medical condition requires that you take high doses of pregnenolone, have your doctor prescribe you a few pills of a beta-blocker such as propranolol to carry with you in case you suddenly develop a palpitation.

Recommendations

Preg is a fascinating hormone and there's still a great deal we need to learn about its potential. Eventually it could be found to play a role, either by itself or with other natural supplements, in arthritis therapy, seizure control, intelligence enhancement, and a number of medical and psychiatric conditions. Caution is advised until we learn more. Keep your dosage level to a minimum. See the end of the chapter for guidelines.

MELATONIN: NATURE'S SLEEPING PILL

Melatonin is a hormone made in the pineal gland, a small, pea-sized gland located in the middle of the brain. This hormone is released at night and helps us get a deeper sleep. Cognitive improvements can occur when the proper use of melatonin improves sleep patterns and provides a deeper, more restful sleep.

Jerry, a sixty-eight-year-old retired policeman, says,

> I've had difficulty sleeping most of my adult life since work schedules kept changing. Sometimes I would do the night shift for a month and then switch to day shift. I think getting older made things worse, too. I find melatonin helps me tremendously. I take about 0.5 mg two or three nights a week. I sleep better, have more energy during the day, and feel more rested. I really like melatonin. I wish I knew about it years ago.

Health Claims

Melatonin became very popular in 1996 because of media reports that, in addition to treating insomnia, melatonin could prolong life, act as an antioxidant, prevent tumors, improve sex, and treat jet lag. Are any of these claims true?

A review of the published studies, and my clinical experience, indicates that melatonin works well as a sleep aid, does not improve sex drive, works well for jet lag, and can slightly improve mood by providing a deep sleep at night. No long-term human studies are available to indicate whether regular use prolongs life. A few trials have indicated melatonin also has antitumor potential. Laboratory studies have indicated melatonin to have antioxidant properties protecting brain cells from damage (Skaper 1998). Whether melatonin does so in the human body in the dosages normally consumed for sleep is not known.

Availability and Dosage

Melatonin is sold in regular pills, sublingual lozenges, under-the-tongue liquid, time-release tablets or capsules, and even in a tea form. Dosages sold usually range from 0.3 to 3 mg. The time-release form is a good option and provides more consistent sleep throughout the night.

The Author's Experience

I have personally taken 0.3 to 1 mg of melatonin once or twice a week since 1995. Melatonin improves my sleeping patterns. But if I use it frequently, I notice the development of tolerance. (The serotonin precursor 5-HTP has sleep-inducing properties similar to melatonin.)

Cautions and Side Effects

Amounts greater than 0.5 mg can produce vivid dreams, including nightmares. Even higher amounts can cause morning grogginess and lethargy. Nightly use in high dosages for prolonged periods may lead to temporary loss of sexual interest and low mood. Melatonin is very safe, however, when used appropriately.

Recommendations

Until more research is available, limit dosage to 0.3 to 1 mg. It can be taken a half hour to two hours before bed, preferably on an empty stomach. The time-release form is a good option. Small doses of melatonin can be combined with valerian, hops, and other sedative herbs.

Melatonin should not be used regularly for more than two nights a week, due to the possible induction of tolerance, and the effects are unknown when used nightly for prolonged periods.

THE MULTI-HORMONE REPLACEMENT SOLUTION

Many questions remain unanswered as to whether hormone replacement in middle-aged and older individuals is a proper medical approach to fighting the neuronal degeneration and cognitive decline that occurs with the aging process. I am certain that debate in this area will continue for a long time. It's quite likely that we'll eventually find that hormone replacement will benefit certain individuals but the required dosages may be much lower than are currently recommended. It may turn out that the best hormone-replacement regimen involves giving a small amount of Preg, DHEA, and perhaps testosterone to men, and Preg, DHEA, and estrogens (and progesterone?) to women. On the downside, it's possible that regular, high-dose hormone use could increase the risk of cancer in certain individuals.

Following are some guidelines on hormone-replacement therapy. Please discuss these with your physician if you're planning to take hormones on a regular basis. I wish to emphasize that these are suggestions only, and in no way do I propose that these dosages are right for everyone. Everyone has a unique biochemistry. Some may not need any of these hormones, while others may benefit from them. Also, your health-care provider may have a different opinion, believing that the following recommendations are too low, too high, or perhaps inappropriate for you.

DO YOU NEED PHYSICAL EXAMS AND TESTS?

Your health-care provider should be consulted anytime you plan to regularly use hormone supplements. Taking hormones is not as simple as popping a multivitamin pill.

Following are some evaluations that should be considered while you're on long-term hormone-replacement therapy. Both you and your health-care practitioner need to be involved. These are just guidelines and you may consider having more or less done, depending on your particular circumstance. Remember that steroid hormones influence, or are metabolized in, a variety of body tissues including the liver, fat cells, skin, endometrium, myometrium, intestines, breast, kidney, lung, muscle, heart, brain, prostate, testes, ovaries, eyes, and others.

The Basics

Your health-care provider should give you a comprehensive medical examination, inclusive of the areas of weight, blood pressure, heart rate and rhythm, muscle mass, body fat, eyes and vision, hearing, skin (particularly for hair growth, moisture, and pimples), hair (facial and scalp), and brain functions such as mood, alertness, memory, motivation, and sleep patterns. Men should have their prostate glands evaluated routinely. Women need to have regular breast and pelvic exams.

Lab tests

You will probably need a routine urinalysis, along with a blood panel that includes blood count, white count, kidney function, blood sugar, triglycerides, cholesterol, liver enzymes, and thyroid tests.

If the above are not enough to provide the necessary monitoring, your health-care practitioner may order more extensive testing.

READER NOTE: By "hormone holidays," I mean that you go off the hormones once in a while. How often you take off, and for how long, is a decision you can make in consultation with your health-care practitioner. One reasonable approach is to take off one week or two weeks a month, or to take them every other day, or every third day. I recommend that you take hormones in the morning or before noon since taking them later in the day can lead to excessive alertness and insomnia. This is particularly true if you take a high dose.

Men—Ages 40 to 50

Melatonin: 0.2 to 0.5 mg once or twice per week, an hour or two before bedtime, especially if you have difficulty sleeping.

Preg: 1 to 4 mg every other day, frequently taking hormone holidays.

Or

DHEA: 1 to 4 mg every other day, frequently taking hormone holidays.

(**Or** the combination of Preg and DHEA, not exceeding 4 mg every other day, along with frequent hormone holidays.)

Men—Ages 50 to 65

Melatonin: 0.2 to 1 mg once or twice a week an hour or so before bedtime, especially if you have difficulty sleeping.

Preg: 1 to 5 mg every other day, frequently taking hormone holidays.

Or

DHEA: 1 to 5 mg every other day, frequently taking hormone holidays.

(**Or** the combination of Preg and DHEA, not exceeding 5 mg every other day, along with hormone holidays.)

Men—Ages 65 and Older

Melatonin: 0.3 to 1 mg one to three times per week, an hour or so before bedtime, especially if you have difficulty sleeping.

Preg: 1 to 6 mg every other day, occasionally taking hormone holidays.

Or

DHEA: 1 to 6 mg every other day, occasionally taking hormone holidays.

(**Or** the combination of Preg and DHEA, not exceeding 6 mg every other day, with hormone holidays.)

Testosterone: Optional, if DHEA by itself does not provide enough of an androgenic effect.

Premenopausal Women—Ages 40 to About 50

Melatonin: 0.2 to 0.5 mg once or twice per week, an hour or two before bedtime, especially if you have difficulty sleeping.

Preg: 1 to 3 mg every other day, frequently taking hormone holidays.

Or

DHEA: 1 to 3 mg every other day, frequently taking hormone holidays.

(**Or** the combination of Preg and DHEA, not exceeding 3 mg every other day, with hormone holidays.)

Postmenopausal Women—Ages 50 to 65

Melatonin: 0.2 to 1 mg once or twice a week, an hour or so before bedtime, especially if you have difficulty sleeping.

Preg: 1 to 4 mg every other day, occasionally taking hormone holidays.

Or

DHEA: 1 to 4 mg every other day, occasionally taking hormone holidays.

(**Or** the combination of Preg and DHEA, not exceeding 4 mg every other day, with hormone holidays.)

Estrogen: Generally half to a third of the dose normally recommended; for instance, in the case of Premarin, 0.2 to 0.3 mg would be adequate, instead of 0.625. Since DHEA gets partially converted into female hormones, women taking DHEA would need to reduce their dosage of estrogens.*

Women—Ages 65 and Over

Melatonin: 0.3 to 1 mg once, twice, or three times per week, an hour or so before bedtime, especially if you have difficulty sleeping.

Preg: 1 to 5 mg every other day, occasionally taking hormone holidays.

Or

DHEA: 1 to 5 mg every other day, occasionally taking hormone holidays.

(**Or** the combination of Preg and DHEA, not exceeding 5 mg every other day, with hormone holidays.)

Estrogen: See recommendations above.

Progesterone: See recommendations below.**

---

* I recommend natural or plant estrogens instead of the synthetic versions or those collected from urine (Premarin). Synthetic versions and Premarin are available by prescription only. I also recommend you consume between one and four ounces of a soy product a day. This could be in the form of tofu, soymilk, or another form. Increasing soy intake or taking soy extracts could reduce the need for estrogen.

** **Progesterone:** Since Preg converts into progesterone, the use of Preg makes the need for progesterone less essential. If you do take progesterone, use the natural form in micronized, sublingual, or cream forms. You will need a much lower dose of progesterone if you're already on Preg since many of their effects overlap. Progesterone, in the appropriate strength, is available by prescription. Low-dose progesterone creams are also sold over-the-counter.

I believe in synergism, the use of low doses of many nutrients and hormones instead of a high dose of just one. For instance, instead of taking a high dose of Preg, such as 10 mg, I prefer someone take 1 to 3 mg but, in addition, supplement with some of the other nutrients discussed in this book.

Summary

I believe that with the right dosage and mix of hormone supplements, some individuals can improve the quality of their lives and enhance mental function. The trick is to find the right combination, frequency, and dosages while minimizing potential side effects.

It will take us decades to learn the long-term effects of different hormone supplements and their combinations. In the meantime, many of these hormones are readily available over-the-counter, and people want guidelines.

- If you plan to take these hormones, err on the side of taking less, not more. Take hormone holidays. Please keep in mind that the dosages available over-the-counter are often too high and you may need to take only a tiny fraction of these pills. Have a health-care provider monitor you closely.

FIFTEEN

Psychoactive Herbs—Recommended by Mother Nature

I was trained at Thomas Jefferson Medical School, a very conservative institution located in Philadelphia. During my four-year medical education in the early 1980s, I don't recall any of my teachers ever mentioning nutritional or herbal therapies. I graduated from medical school truly believing that if there *were* any effective herbal remedies, our teachers would have discussed them. Years later, when I first started reading on my own about the potential uses of herbs for the treatment of medical and psychiatric conditions, I was skeptical. But over the past few years of studying herbs, reviewing the research, taking them myself, and prescribing them to patients, I must say that I'm now a convert. Many herbs have very interesting compounds that have significant effects on the body and brain. In fact, there are countless chemicals found in herbs, and some of them are as powerful as pharmaceutical medicines.

Unfortunately, due to the fact that the natural chemicals in plants cannot be patented, funding for research with herbs has been slow. Only a few, such as St. John's wort, saw palmetto, kava, ginseng, and ginkgo, have undergone extensive human trials. In this chapter I present some common herbs that you probably have read about, and also discuss some herbs imported from Asia and South America that seem to have an effect on brain function. The field of herbal medicine fascinates me since there are countless undiscovered chemicals within herbs that eventually could be found to have a therapeutic role in medical and psychiatric conditions. There are thousands of herbs and herbal combinations developed by healers from Asia, Africa, and South America. With time, many of these will find their way into North America and Europe.

A common term you will come across when reviewing herbs in this section is the word *adaptogen.* This is a nonspecific word indicating that the herb historically has been found to have several positive properties, particularly in increasing energy and improving resistance to stress and disease.

What Can Psychoactive Herbs Do for You?

There are thousands of different chemicals within herbs, and generalizations cannot be made regarding their effects on the brain. There's a significant overlap in the cognitive effects of various herbs, but they can be loosely categorized in the following ways:

- Herbs that increase energy—these include the adaptogens ginseng, maca, and schisandra, and certain foodlike extracts such as royal jelly.
- Herbs that are particularly useful for anxiety disorders—kava is the most effective, although some of the adaptogens also work well. Ashwagandha and reishi are good options, too.
- Herbs that improve memory—ginkgo is the most well studied herb in this category although bacopa, huperzine A, and vinpocetine can be helpful.
- Herbs that improve mood—St. John's wort is the most consistent mood-elevating herb, although others have mild-to-moderate mood-elevating properties.
- Herbs that improve sex drive—many herbs, such as ginseng, have

been promoted to have aphrodisiac qualities, but studies are limited. My clinical experience indicates ashwagandha is a good libido-enhancing herb.

ASHWAGANDHA *(WITHANIA SOMNIFERA)*

Ashwagandha is a shrub cultivated in India and North America; the roots have been used for thousands of years by Ayurvedic practitioners as a folk remedy. It contains flavonoids and several active ingredients of the withanolide class (Elsakka 1990). Several studies over the past few years have indicated that ashwagandha has antioxidant properties and influences brain chemistry.

Researchers from Banaras Hindu University in Varanasi, India, have discovered that some of the chemicals within this herb are powerful antioxidants (Bhattacharya 1997). They tested these compounds for their effects on rat brains and found an increase in the levels of three natural antioxidants—superoxide dismutase, catalase, and glutathione peroxidase. They say, "These findings are consistent with the therapeutic use of *W. somnifera* as an Ayurvedic rasayana (health promoter). The antioxidant effect of active principles of *W. somnifera* may explain, at least in part, the reported anti-stress, cognition-facilitating, anti-inflammatory and anti-aging effects produced by them in experimental animals, and in clinical situations." Another study has confirmed that extracts from ashwagandha have antioxidant properties (Dhuley 1998).

Ashwagandha may affect brain chemistry; it is used in India to treat mental deficits in geriatric patients, including amnesia. Researchers from the University of Leipzig in Germany wanted to find out which neurotransmitters were influenced by ashwagandha (Schliebs 1997). After injecting some of the chemicals in ashwagandha into rats, the researchers later examined slices of the rats' brains and found an increase in acetylcholine receptor activity.The researchers say, "The drug-induced increase in acetylcholine receptor capacity might partly explain the cognition-enhancing and memory-improving effects of extracts from *Withania somnifera* observed in animals and humans."

A study done in 1991 at the Department of Pharmacology, University of Texas Health Science Center, indicated that extracts of ashwagandha had GABA-like activity (Mehta 1991). This may account for this herb's antianxiety effects.

Availability and Dosage

Ashwagandha is sold in capsules of 500 mg, and is available as a dried root, powder, or liquid extract. It is often combined with other herbs.

Expert Opinions

Dr. Shailinder Sodhi, N.D., an expert in Ayurvedic medicine from Bellevue, Washington, says, "Ashwagandha provides a sense of well-being with a decrease in anxiety. Users feel mellow. It is also a good aphrodisiac. Lise Alschuler, N.D., Chair of the Botanical Medicine Department at Bastyr University in Seattle, Washington, adds, "My clinical experience indicates that ashwagandha reduces anxiety and is helpful for insomnia. I recommend it for patients who are tense and need a calming herb. They can think more clearly after being relaxed."

The Author's Experience

I tried ashwagandha pills at a dose of 500 mg each at breakfast and lunch for a week. It made me calm and sleepy, and I am quite certain that it also increased my interest in sex. I find ashwagandha is better suited for me to take in the evening due to its sedative effects.

Recommendations

Ashwagandha is an excellent herb for individuals who are tense and anxious, particularly if they suffer a loss of interest in sex. Taking this herb is in the evening is a good option since it can induce sleepiness in some people. However, if you have daytime anxiety or you are tense, you can take it at breakfast or lunchtime.

GINKGO BILOBA

Extracts from the leaves of the ginkgo biloba tree have been used therapeutically in China for millennia. According to fossil records, the ginkgo tree has been around for over 200 million years and is one of the oldest still-existing tree species on earth. Individual trees live up to one thousand years. Ginkgo, like ginseng, is mentioned in the traditional Chinese pharmacopoeia. Ginkgo extracts are among the most widely studied and prescribed drugs in Europe to alleviate symptoms associated with a wide range of conditions. The main indications for these extracts are peripheral vascular disease and the therapy of age-related cognitive decline. Ginkgo contains many different substances, but most of them fall into two main categories: *flavonoids* and *terpene lactones*.

Flavonoids are natural substances that are also found in fruits and vegetables (see Chapter 11). Flavonoids act as antioxidants, have an influence on the immune system, and interfere with tumor formation. Ginkgo contains many flavonoids, but the most concentrated are kaempferol, quercetin, and isorhamnetin. Most ginkgo products on the market list a flavonoid concentration of 24 percent—you will often see "24%" printed on packages or bottles of ginkgo. Terpene lactones are what give ginkgo a bitter and strong flavor. The most important terpenes are the ginkgolides and bilobides. Ginkgolides have not yet been found in any other living plant species.

At least two-thirds of individuals I have treated or interviewed have noticed positive benefits from ginkgo. Gerry, a seventy-seven-year-old retired postal worker, says, "Ginkgo has helped my tinnitus [ringing in the ears]. It also works very well in keeping me alert and focused. I take 60 mg for breakfast and lunch." Mandy, a sixty-six-year-old actress, likes the effect of this herb. She reports, "I've been taking gingko for about four months now, and the improvement in my memory function is so much better I wouldn't even consider not taking it now."

However, not everyone notices benefits. Sandra, a thirty-seven-year-old, is disappointed. She says, "I took ginkgo for a period of six months after I heard all the positive benefits that other people were experiencing. Frankly, I haven't noticed any major difference."

How Does Ginkgo Work?

The active ingredients in gingko are believed to produce their beneficial effects by acting as antioxidants, preventing red blood cells and platelets from aggregating to form clots, allowing more oxygen to reach neurons, and improving circulation in tiny blood vessels by inducing relaxation of the muscles surrounding blood vessels. Even circulation to the eyes improves when subjects are given ginkgo (Chung 1999).

Clinical Uses

The primary indications for ginkgo use are age-related cognitive decline (ARCD) and Alzheimer's disease.

Age-related cognitive decline is a term that describes a collection of symptoms; these include difficulty in concentration and memory, absentmindedness, confusion, lack of mental energy, and, sometimes, depressive mood. Some of these symptoms may be associated with not enough blood reaching the brain, hence a potential justification for the use of gingko in lessening these symptoms. Ginkgo improves communication between nerve cells and enhances blood flow to the brain. It is licensed in Germany for the treatment of ARCD. Ginkgo may have promise in the treatment of Parkinson's disease and Alzheimer's when used together with other conventional medicines. A well-publicized study in the *Journal of the American Medical Association* indicated that 120 mg of ginkgo extract per day for one year was able to slightly improve cognitive performance in patients with Alzheimer's disease (Le Bars 1997).

What Dosages Are Best?

The majority of the studies done thus far with ginkgo have used daily dosages of 120 to 160 mg (50:1 concentration, 24% flavonoids). Patients generally took 40 mg three to four times a day. Treatment may be needed for a few weeks before positive results can be fully appreciated. Most manufacturers sell pills that contain 40 or 60 mg of ginkgo.

You may wish to start with one or two pills a day to see if there is any improvement in memory or thinking. Ginkgo is best taken early in the day, and no later than afternoon.

The Author's Experience

I have found that I think more clearly and faster, and am slightly more alert and talkative when I use gingko. The effects, though, are subtle.

Cautions and Side Effects

No serious side effects have been noted in formal studies with ginkgo. In rare cases, mild stomach or intestinal complaints, headache, and allergic skin reactions have been reported. There have been rare mentions of internal bleeding when ginkgo was combined with other blood thinners such as aspirin or coumadin. Ginkgo has antiplatelet activity and hence can prolong the time it takes to form a blood clot.

Recommendations

Ginkgo appears to be useful in memory loss due to aging or Alzheimer's disease. Because of its antioxidant properties, it may be useful in individuals with cerebrovascular disease. Due to its blood-thinning properties, a dose of 60 mg a day should not be exceeded on a long-term daily basis unless a health-care provider monitors you. Keep in mind that other nutrients and drugs have blood-thinning properties, including coumadin, aspirin, fish oils, and vinpocetine.

GINSENG

The root of the ginseng plant has been used in China, Japan, and Korea for many centuries in the therapy of psychiatric and neurological disorders. There are several varieties of ginseng sold over-the-counter: Asian ginseng (*Panax ginseng*), American ginseng (*Panax quinquefolius*), and Siberian ginseng (*Eleutherococcus chinensis*) are the most common. Technically, Siberian ginseng does not belong in the same genus as Asian or American ginseng and does not contain the same ingredients. As a rule, Chinese ginseng is more stimulating and raises body temperature while American ginseng is less heating and less stimulating. Siberian ginseng is neutral. Hundreds of ginseng products are available over-the-counter in different doses and combinations.

The roots of Chinese and American ginseng contain several saponins named ginsenosides that are believed to contribute to the adaptogenic properties. They are used in traditional Chinese medicine to improve stamina and combat fatigue and stress. Saponins are interesting natural compounds found in many plants, herbs, roots, and beans. Saponins have potential in the prevention and treatment of diseases of the heart and circulatory system (Purmova 1995). For instance, they inhibit the formation of lipid peroxides (fat oxidation) in cardiac muscle or in the liver; they decrease blood coagulation, cholesterol, and sugar levels in blood; and they stimulate the immune system. Some saponins may even have antitumor properties (Wakabayashi 1998).

The biochemical mechanisms of ginseng remain unclear, although there is extensive literature that deals with its effects on the brain (memory, learning, and behavior), neuroendocrine function, carbohydrate and lipid metabolism, immune function, and the cardiovascular system. Reports are often contradictory, perhaps because the ginsenoside content of ginseng root or root extracts can differ—depending on the species, method of extraction, subsequent treatment, or even the season of collection.

Most patients who take ginseng notice an improvement in energy, vitality, feelings of well-being, and mental clarity.

Laboratory and Human Studies

Let's examine some of the studies done with ginseng:

- **Cognitive functioning:** Various tests of mental performance were carried out in a group of sixteen healthy male volunteers given a standardized preparation of Asian ginseng (100 mg twice a day for twelve weeks, of a product called G-115). A similar group was given identical placebo capsules under double-blind conditions (D'Angelo 1986). A favorable effect of ginseng was observed in attention, mental arithmetic, logical deduction, and auditory reaction time.

  Researchers at Cognitive Drug Research Ltd., Beech Hill, Reading, England, evaluated the effects of a ginkgo biloba/ginseng combination on cognitive function (Wesnes 1997). The study lasted ninety days and was performed in a double-blind, placebo-controlled manner with sixty-four healthy volunteers (aged 40 to 65 years) who had mild fatigue and low mood. There were improvements noted in memory and overall cognitive functioning. The treatment was well tolerated by all volunteers.

  Ginseng root saponin at a dose of 50 mg three times a day, was given for two months to 358 middle-aged and elderly individuals (Zhao 1990). The results showed that the herb improved memory and immunity.
- **Diabetes and mood:** To investigate the effect of ginseng on newly diagnosed noninsulin-dependent diabetes mellitus (NIDDM) patients, thirty NIDDM patients were treated for eight weeks with ginseng extract (100 or 200 mg) or placebo in a double-blind placebo-controlled manner (Sotaniemi 1995). The results showed ginseng therapy elevated mood, improved psychophysical performance, and reduced fasting blood glucose.
- **Quality of life:** The aim of this study was to compare the quality-of-life parameters in subjects receiving multivitamins plus ginseng, with those found in subjects receiving multivitamins alone (Caso Marasco 1996). The study was randomized and

double-blind, and it involved 625 patients of both sexes divided into two groups taking one capsule per day for twelve weeks. Group A received vitamins, minerals, trace elements, and ginseng extract, while group B received vitamins, minerals, and trace elements only. By the end of the study, both group A and group B tested positively on a questionnaire evaluating quality of life, but group A had a higher score.

Availability and Dosage

Countless varieties and dosages of ginseng are available. One option is to buy a product that has a standardized extract of 3 to 7 percent ginsenosides. Use 100 mg of this extract in the morning a few times a week. You may require 500 to 2000 mg of crude extracts to feel the effects. It's best to cycle the use of ginseng. For instance, you can take it for two or three weeks and then take off a few weeks.

An Expert's Opinion

Lise Alschuler, N.D., Chair of the Botanical Medicine Department at Bastyr University in Seattle, Washington, says, "My favorite adaptogen is Siberian ginseng. I take it myself and recommend it to patients. I normally take it for a few weeks or months and then go off it for an extended period. This herb enhances well-being, increases alertness, decreases anxiety, and provides more energy.

The Author's Experience

The effects from ginseng are subtle but definitely present. I have tried Asian ginseng on numerous occasions. I notice an enhancement in alertness, motivation, focus, and mood, along with a sense of peacefulness. The effects seem to improve on subsequent days of use. High doses interfere with sleep.

Cautions and Side Effects

Insomnia is a common side effect from ginseng overuse, particularly with Asian ginseng—especially when it's combined in high doses with other herbs or nutrients that cause alertness. Althea, a thirty-eight-year-old owner of a garden shop in Maui, says,

> I tried taking a combination of kava and American ginseng that was recommended by a Chinese physician for fatigue. I took it for two weeks. I felt really better emotionally, mellow, and with increased energy. Then I started to have increased sleep problems and insomnia. I went three days being so mentally and physically overstimulated that I hardly got any sleep. I imagine this is what being on 'speed' must feel like. I stopped taking the herbs, and within two days I slowly returned to my normal state.

This story confirms my recommendation in Chapter 2 that dosages of nutrients and herbs have to be constantly evaluated since they can build up in the system cumulatively.

Recommendations

Many people who take ginseng find this herb to be a good overall energizer and cognitive enhancer. Due to the tremendous variety of products sold, it is difficult to give definite dosage recommendations. You could certainly try a few products to see which one(s) give you a positive effect. In practical and simple terms, Asian ginseng raises body temperature and is more stimulating, while American ginseng is more cooling and calming. The effects of Siberian ginseng fall somewhere between these two. See this chapter's summary for additional recommendations.

HUPERZINE A

Huperzine A is an extract from a club moss (*Huperzia serrata*) that has been used for centuries in Chinese folk medicine. Its action has been attributed to its ability to strongly inhibit acetylcholinesterase, the enzyme that breaks down acetylcholine in the synaptic cleft (see Chapter 4).

Acetylcholine is involved in memory and learning. By inhibiting the enzyme that breaks it down, more acetylcholine becomes available to stimulate neurons. Alzheimer's disease is a condition where there's a relative shortage of acetylcholine.

Several studies have been done over the past few years with huperzine A, both in China and the United States. These studies have shown that huperzine A is many times more effective and selective than tacrine (a cholinesterase-inhibiting pharmaceutical drug) in inhibiting cholinesterase (Cheng 1996). Huperzine A has also been found to be beneficial in patients with Alzheimer's disease. Scientists at Zhejiang Medical University, in Hangzhou, China, administered 0.2 mg of huperzine A to fifty patients with Alzheimer's disease for a period of eight weeks and compared the results to a group who received placebo pills (Xu 1995). The study was done in a double-blind, placebo-controlled, and randomized manner. The results showed 58 percent of the patients treated with huperzine A had improvements in memory, cognition, and behavioral functions whereas only 36 percent of those on placebo improved. No severe side effects were found. Blood pressure, heart rate, electrocardiogram, electroencephalogram, and liver and urine tests did not show any major abnormalities. The researchers say, "Huperzine A is a promising drug for symptomatic treatment of Alzheimer's disease."

This club-moss extract may also benefit older individuals with dementia. A study was conducted with fifty-six patients suffering from multi-infarct dementia (multiple small strokes) and one hundred patients with senile memory disorders (Zhang 1991). The dose used for multi-infarct dementia was 0.05 mg twice a day for four weeks, whereas that for senile memory disorders was 0.03 mg twice a day for two weeks. Most patients had an improvement in memory. A few reported slight dizziness, but this did not affect the therapeutic effects.

Huperzine was even mentioned in the *Journal of the American Medical Association* as a possible herbal therapy for Alzheimer's disease (Skolnick 1997).

Availability and Dosage
Huperzine A is sold either by itself in doses of 0.05 mg, or in lower doses combined with other mind-boosting nutrients.

The Author's Experience
I took a capsule containing 50 micrograms (0.05 mg) of huperzine A in the morning, at nine A.M. on an empty stomach. Within an hour I could feel a subtle effect. This consisted mostly of feeling slightly more alert and focused. Over the next hour I took two additional capsules and then ate breakfast. My focus and concentration were slightly improved all day long and well into the evening. It didn't seem that huperzine A had any effect on mood, libido, or appetite. No side effects occurred.

One study has shown that huperzine A is absorbed rapidly when taken orally, distributed widely in the body, and eliminated at a moderate rate (Qian 1995). This rapid absorption and moderate elimination is consistent with my observation of the effects within an hour and the continuation of the effects late into the evening.

Recommendations
Huperzine A appears to be a promising alternative to cholinesterase-inhibitor drugs used in Alzheimer's disease. More studies are required to determine its long-term safety and side-effect profile. Until we learn more about this herbal extract, I recommend its use only in the therapy of AD, and only under medical supervision.

KAVA *(PIPER METHYSTICUM)*

More than 20 million Americans suffer from anxiety disorders, and countless others experience everyday stress. Since stress can interfere with mental clarity, the occasional use of kava can provide cognitive benefits.

Kava is a plant grown in the South Pacific Islands; the roots have been used by Polynesians as a psychoactive agent for centuries. The root of the kava plant contains a variety of chemicals known as kavalactones. Specific names for some of these kavalactones include kawain, dihydrokawain, methysticin, and yangonin. Kavalactones influence a number of the brain receptors involved in relaxation and mental clarity.

Until 1997, only a few short-term placebo-controlled studies on kava extract ingestion had been published. In 1997, Dr. Hans-Peter Volz, from the Department of Psychiatry, Jena University, in Jena, Germany, published the results of the longest comprehensive human trial yet, which used extracts of kava in 101 patients. All of the patients suffered from anxiety and tension. Many had a fear of public places (agoraphobia), social phobia, generalized anxiety disorder, and adjustment disorder with anxiety. The dosage given was one capsule three times a day, of 70 mg of kavalactones. The study lasted twenty-five weeks, and the results showed that the effectiveness of kava was superior to that of placebo. The specific areas that were improved included anxious mood, tension, and fears. Patients tolerated kava well, and adverse reactions were rare.

The Kava Experience

Not everyone reacts exactly the same way to this herb, because each one of us has a different biochemistry. Furthermore, different products on the market may have different amounts or constituents of kavalactones within them.

Most of the time, the effects of kava are noticed within an hour or two and can last several hours. If you are already relaxed and have no muscle tension, you won't notice the calming effects of kava as much as someone who is anxious. Following are some common feelings that most users report; I have personally experienced these effects.

- A state of relaxation without interference in mental acuity, at least for the first few hours. Whether you feel more alert or sleepy from kava ingestion will depend on your individual biochemistry, and also from the product you are using. Often there's a feeling of alertness, followed by being drowsy and sleepy hours later. Many people have the misconception that kava is a sedative that will make one feel sleepy right away. In most cases the sedation follows an initial period of alertness.

- Less muscle tension.
- Feelings of peacefulness and contentment with mild euphoria.
- A few report a slight, temporary enhancement of visual acuity. Objects and people take on a sharper look.

The fact that kava causes relaxation, while keeping one mentally alert, distinguishes it from many drugs used for anxiety (such as Xanax and Valium), since these drugs have a tendency to interfere markedly with cognitive functioning.

Availability and Dosage

Kava is sold in a number of dosages and forms. A dose of 70 to 100 mg of kavalactones once or twice a day can be helpful in cases of anxiety. Try at least two or three different products before drawing an opinion about kava's effectiveness.

Recommendations

Kava is an excellent herb to use occasionally in order to relieve tension and stress. Many users find it to be a good alternative to antianxiety drugs. For more details, see my book *Kava: The Miracle Antianxiety Herb.*

The best time to take kava is in the late afternoon or early evening, unless you are very anxious during the day in which case you can take it in the morning or midday. Some individuals may need higher doses to notice an effect.

ST. JOHN'S WORT *(HYPERICUM PERFORATUM)*

This simple herb took the media spotlight in 1997. What propelled St. John's wort to the status of superstar herbal antidepressant was a study published in the *British Medical Journal* (Linde 1996); the study was entitled "St. John's wort for depression—an overview and meta-analysis of randomized clinical trials." The reason this study garnered such media attention was that it was a *meta-analysis*, meaning the authors thoroughly reviewed twenty-three previous studies published on this herb and pooled the results together. Most of these studies were published in foreign journals, and had not attracted the attention of the mainstream American media. This herb has been popular in Germany and many other European countries for decades, prescribed more often than pharmaceutical antidepressants.

The overall interpretation of this meta-analysis showed that St. John's wort was significantly superior to placebo and was as effective as pharmaceutical antidepressants—and with fewer side effects. More than half of the patients on prescription antidepressant drugs reported side effects, compared to less than 20 percent of those taking the herb.

Extracts from this herb contain a number of groups of compounds, including hypericins and flavonoids. Many of the available preparations of St. John's wort are standardized, based on the hypericin content and not necessarily on the flavonoids.

How Does it Work?

Since there are a quite a number of compounds within St. John's wort extract, it has been difficult to determine the precise ways this herb works in relieving depression. Some studies indicate this herb influences brain-chemical levels, such as dopamine, serotonin, and norepinephrine.

Most of my patients who have taken St. John's wort have noticed a sense of well-being, more alertness and energy, and an end to feelings of procrastination. There is a motivation to get things done, such as work projects and housecleaning. Some patients also report having a greater interest in being social and interacting with friends, and meeting new people.

It may take one or two weeks to notice the antidepressant effects. I recommend you take the herb for at least one month before forming an opinion on its effectiveness.

Availability and Dosage

Most of the extracts you purchase over-the-counter contain 0.3 percent hypericins in a 300-mg dose because they are based on a European formulation that has been used as the standard in the various studies conducted over the years.

Many of the studies evaluating the effectiveness of St. John's wort have used a dosage of 300 mg of the extract three times a day. I find that patients experience a higher rate of insomnia when they take three pills a day. Start with one pill in the morning. If there has been no improvement after a few days, add a second pill with lunch. Every person has a unique biochemistry. Some may find that one pill in the morning, or even one every other morning, is adequate, while others may require three pills a day. If you have only a mild case of depression, I recommend you start with just one pill before increasing the dosage. (See Chapter 19 on how to use St. John's wort in combination with other mood-elevating nutrients.)

The Author's Experience

I notice the effects of this herb, such as an enhanced sense of well-being, the very first day of taking it, but the effects become more pronounced over the next few days of use. I experience insomnia when my dosage exceeds two pills a day.

Cautions and Side Effects

Fortunately, St. John's wort has few side effects. The side effects reported in scientific studies include dizziness, nausea, tiredness, restlessness, dry mouth, and allergic reactions, including hives or itching; in most studies, these occurred in less than 10 percent of users. These side effects are dose-dependent, meaning lower dosages would minimize any potential negative outcomes. It's very rare to have side effects while taking a daily dose of 300 mg for less than two months.

It's best to avoid excessive sun exposure while taking St. John's wort due to possible skin reactions.

Recommendations

St. John's wort is definitely a good antidepressant and an effective alternative to pharmaceutical antidepressants in cases of mild-to-moderate depression.

Most cases of depression last only a few months. I advise that this herb be used continuously for no longer than six months. We don't have long-term studies to know what kind of influence this herb has on our bodies. If the depression returns, then this medicine can be restarted. The majority of the human trials with this herb have lasted less than three months.

VINPOCETINE

Vinpocetine is chemically related to, and derived from, vincamine, an alkaloid found in the periwinkle plant. Vinpocetine became available over-the-counter in 1998. It was introduced into clinical practice in Europe more than two decades ago for the treatment of cerebrovascular disorders and related symptoms. Experiments with vinpocetine indicate that it can dilate blood vessels, enhance circulation in the brain, improve oxygen utilization, make red blood cells more pliable, and inhibit aggregation of platelets (Kiss 1996). Vinpocetine may even have antioxidant properties (Orvisky 1997).

There have been quite a few studies with vinpocetine. Researchers at the University of Surrey in Guildford, England, administered vinpocetine to patients suffering from mild-to-moderate dementia (Hindmarch 1991). Two hundred and three patients included in a placebo-controlled, randomized double-blind trial received every day for sixteen weeks either 10 mg doses of vinpocetine three times a day, 20 mg doses of vinpocetine three times a day, or placebo three times a day. There were no clinically relevant side effects reported. Statistically significant cognitive improvements were found in favor of active treatment groups compared to placebo. The patients on 10 mg performed slightly better than those on 20 mg.

Fifteen Alzheimer patients were treated with increasing doses of vinpocetine (30, 45, and 60 mg per day) in an open-label pilot trial during a one-year period (Thal 1989). The study was done at Veterans Administration Medical Center, in San Diego, California. Vinpocetine failed to improve cognition at any dose tested. There were no significant side effects from the therapy.

In a double-blind clinical trial, vinpocetine was shown to offer significant improvement in elderly patients with chronic cerebral dysfunction (Balestreri 1987). Forty-two patients received 10 mg of vinpocetine three times a day for thirty days, then 5 mg three times a day for sixty days. Matching placebo tablets were given to another forty patients for the ninety-day trial period. Patients on vinpocetine scored consistently better in all cognitive evaluations. No serious side effects were reported.

Twelve healthy female volunteers received pre-treatments with vinpocetine 40 mg three times a day or placebo for two days according to a randomized double-blind crossover design (Subhan 1985). On the third day of treatment, and one hour following morning dosage, subjects completed a battery of psychological tests. Memory was significantly improved following treatment with vinpocetine when compared to placebo.

Availability and Dosage

Vinpocetine is sold in 5 and 10 mg pills. Levels peak in the bloodstream within an hour and a half after ingestion.

Users' Experiences

Dennis, a seventy-two-year-old patient with age-related cognitive decline, says, "I take 5 mg of vinpocetine at breakfast and lunch. I feel more focused, and it seems that I can make decisions quicker. I also notice colors to be more vivid." Other patients report similar positive effects.

Dr. Polimeni, in Rome, Italy, says, "Vinpocetine is a good cognitive enhancer. It improves visual and auditory perception similar to pregnenolone. My patients appreciate the effects better after a few days of therapy."

The Author's Experience

I like the effects of vinpocetine. On 10 mg, I notice improvement in concentration and focus, and enhancement of color perception, peaking at about two hours after dosing. Thereafter the effects gradually decrease, but persist for a few hours. I do not notice any significant changes in mood or energy levels.

Cautions and Side Effects

The long-term effects of vinpocetine are not known. It does have blood-thinning potential, hence those taking warfarin or high doses of aspirin or other blood thinners need to inform their physician before use.

Recommendations

Vinpocetine appears to be beneficial in cognitive disorders that are due to poor blood flow to the brain. Therefore individuals with atherosclerotic vascular disease are probably most likely to benefit from vinpocetine. Until long-term studies are available, regular intake for prolonged periods should be limited to 2.5 or 5 mg once or twice daily.

ADDITIONAL HERBS AND FOODLIKE SUPPLEMENTS

There are many herbs that are reputed to influence mental function. A partial list includes (bacopa monniera), cordyceps, gotu kola, rosemary, maca, Fo-ti, reishi, and schisandra. Then there are foodlike supplements such as spirulina, blue-green algae, and royal jelly. The research with many of these supplements is very limited. I am certain that some of them do have an effect since I have personally noticed increased alertness and energy levels when I've taken royal jelly, maca, and gotu kola. I'll just briefly mention a few of these herbs.

- **Bacopa** is an Ayurvedic medicine used in India for memory enhancement, epilepsy, insomnia, and as a mild sedative. This herb commonly grows in marshy areas throughout India. Some studies have shown that bacopa has antioxidant effects (Tripathi 1996), while a study on rats showed bacopa administration improves learning skills (Singh 1982). Bacopa is sold either by itself, or, most commonly, combined with other herbs. Dr. Shailinder Sodhi, an expert in Ayurvedic herbs, reports, "Bacopa is a brain tonic that provides relief from stress; it energizes but does not act as a stimulant. Bacopa is often taken in the morning and the effects can last all day. Users notice alertness, clarity of vision, and stimulation of appetite. The dosage is 125 mg for 50 percent bacosides standardized extract, or 10 ml of the liquid extract." Bacopa has potential as a cognitive aid, but a few more studies are needed in order to determine which neurotransmitters this herb influences and to determine its long-term effectiveness and safety profile.
- **Gotu kola** is an herb commonly used in the Ayurvedic system of medicine. Traditionally gotu kola has been used as a nerve tonic to improve memory and clarity of thinking. It is sold in capsules and in liquid extracts. Most patients notice an increase in alertness and energy. However, a drawback is that it heats the body, so in warm weather you may sweat a little more than usual.

Dr. Sodhi says, "Gotu kola improves circulation, causes alertness, and helps in relaxation. The effects are similar to bacopa but milder."

I've taken gotu kola once at breakfast, four capsules containing 500 mg each. Within a half hour I noticed an increase in alertness and motivation that lasted most of the day. Some people take gotu kola occasionally as a substitute for caffeine in order to be more alert.

- **Maca** is a rootlike vegetable shaped like a radish that grows high in the Andes. Native Peruvians apparently used maca as a food and as medicine. Claims exist that maca is an adaptogen similar to ginseng. Maca has been used traditionally to increase energy and to promote endurance. Maca is available as capsules containing 500 mg of the herb, or as a grain-alcohol extract.

  I've only experimented with maca for a week, with doses ranging from 1000 to 5000 mg. Within a few hours of taking the higher dose of maca, there is an increase in arousal and energy levels. This lasts a few hours and then fades away. There is also a slight mood elevation.
- **Reishi** is a mushroom traditionally used in Asia to help calm the mind, ease tension, improve memory, and sharpen concentration and focus (Teeguarden 1998). Reishi is available as an extract in capsules in a variety of dosages. You will often find it combined with other herbs. Patients report reishi gives them a sense of calmness. Dolores, a forty-four-year old customer-service manager for a major airline, finds this herb helpful. She says, "I'm usually very stressed at work because we get a lot of complaints from customers. When I take reishi, I am able to respond to complaints in a poised and comfortable manner." Rob Underhill, a nutrition educator from Scotts Valley, California, says, "Reishi gives me mental clarity and stamina. It provides a solid base to work from. I feel centered, stable, and can easily access my mental power." Roy Upton, a herbalist from Soquel, California, reports similar effects: "I was burning candles on both ends while traveling,

> giving lectures, and getting little sleep. Reishi helped me stay centered and focused. It gave me a solid physical and mental base to work from without being stimulated. I take up to three tablets a day of 750 mg each."
>
> I've tried a product that contains 600 mg of reishi per capsule. I generally notice the effects when I take two pills. Within a couple of hours, there's a sense of relaxation and calmness, with the urge to take deep, relaxed breaths. My mind stays alert without much sedation or sleepiness. It appears that reishi is an herb that will undoubtedly become more popular with time. It is ideal for individuals who wish to handle stress better and need to stay calm throughout the day. This could apply to office workers, and moms at home taking care of hyperactive children.

With time we are likely to learn more about the effects on the central nervous system of these and many other herbs and foodlike substances.

Recommendations

Following are some practical recommendations for those interested in taking herbs on a regular basis:

- Buy a bottle of one adaptogenic herb such as ginseng or maca and use it regularly for about two weeks. Note how this herb influences you.
- At the end of the two weeks, take a break for a week and purchase another herb. Try this one for two weeks. Again, record your impressions.
- Continue trying the several herbs discussed in this chapter and you'll eventually find out which one(s) you like most.
- Once you've determined the ones that are suitable for you, you can again try each one separately, or you can alternate their use on a daily or weekly basis. It's best not to take these herbs all the

time, but instead to cycle their use. Take a break of a few days when switching from one herb to another.

There are several advantages in alternating the use of different herbs.

1) You'll never find out how much you like the effects of a particular herb if you don't try it.
2) There may be nutrients or compounds within certain other herbs that could be beneficial to you and you will not get exposed to them if you take the same herb all the time.
3) The risk of potential side effects would be minimized. In case your particular body chemistry does not agree with the long-term exposure to a particular herb, alternating them would decrease the chance of an untoward reaction. Some herbs could have potentially toxic or harmful components if used for prolonged periods, but they may not be damaging if your exposure to them is limited.
4) Different herbs will influence different parts of the brain.
5) You may build a tolerance to a certain herb if you take it all the time whereas if you alternate their use, you will continue noticing the cognitive benefits.

It takes time to learn about the different psychoactive herbs and how to best use them for different purposes. I consider learning about these herbs and other mind boosters an exciting, lifelong, enjoyable process.

Summary

As you can see, there are a variety of herbs that have an influence on mood, memory, energy, libido, vision, and cognitive function. How do you decide which one(s) to take?

It's important to differentiate between the herbs that can be taken regularly as adaptogens (such as ginseng) and those that are used for a specific therapeutic purpose. For instance, kava should generally be used if you have stress or anxiety, and St. John's wort is reserved for those with depression. Huperzine A is aimed for those with Alzheimer's disease. Ginkgo improves concentration and memory, and is also recommended for age-related cognitive decline and Alzheimer's disease.

You should also differentiate between the herbs that can cause increased energy, alertness, and warmth—such as Chinese ginseng and gotu kola—and herbs that have a calming effect, such as ashwagandha, kava, and reishi.

PART V

Staying Smart After School

SIXTEEN

The Mind-Boosting Program for Ages 25 to 40

Memory capacity and thinking abilities are excellent during our twenties and thirties. Thus there would be little need to regularly supplement with mind boosters. However, there are occasions when supplements could prove to be beneficial. During this particular life stage, many individuals are attempting to establish a career. Men and women need to be alert and focused at work in order to maximize performance and reap the rewards of accomplishment and success. The appropriate use of mind boosters can help in this regard.

Natural supplements can be helpful in the therapy of mood and anxiety disorders and insomnia. Mood disorders are common in this age group, and depression can certainly interfere with optimal mental functioning. Many natural mood lifters can provide significant assistance, preventing the need for pharmaceutical antidepressants. Alice, a thirty-one-year-old legal assistant, took frequent sick days off work. "I just couldn't make myself get up in the morning and go to work," she lamented. "Even though my boss liked my work, he was about to fire me for being absent so often." After only three weeks' therapy with a combination St. John's wort, B-complex, and CoQ10, Alice's mood brightened and she has rarely missed work since.

Certain supplements can also be helpful in easing the stress and anxiety associated with work and family. Michael, a respiratory therapist at a university hospital, found the occasional use of kava to be significantly helpful in relieving his stress. "I used to have a lot of arguments with the nurses," he recounts. "Since I've started kava, the nurses have commented that I'm much more cheerful and easy to get along with."

A third common problem that interferes with cognition and work performance is insomnia. Sleep difficulties can occur due to stress, lack of physical activity, or anxiety. Many have benefited from the proper use of melatonin, 5-HTP, or certain sleep-inducing herbs such as ashwagandha and hops.

This chapter will provide practical suggestions that address the above issues and will recommend routine supplements for optimal mental functioning.

ROUTINE SUPPLEMENTS FOR THE 25-TO-40 AGE GROUP

Walk into a health-food store or any pharmacy or retail outlet that sells supplements, and you will find shelves and shelves of vitamins, herbs, nutrients, and hormones. Most of these supplements have an effect on the mind. If you're planning to enhance your mental performance, how do you decide which of these supplements are appropriate for you, what dosages you should take, and in what combinations?

There are several factors you need to consider before starting a mind-boosting program. These factors include your age, sex, occupation, lifestyle, diet, medical status, and the potential interaction of these supplements with medicines you may currently be taking.

Please review the top ten mind-boosting principles I discussed in Chapter 2 before you start taking any supplements. I also suggest you follow as many as possible of the dietary and lifestyle recommendations for a healthy mind outlined in Chapter 5. Although it can sometimes be challenging, try to make these recommendations a normal daily habit for the rest of your life. You'll thank yourself many years from now.

If you don't like to take too many pills, I would suggest obtaining many of your basic nutrient needs through a multivitamin complex. There are countless "one-a-day" multivitamin pills you can purchase over-the-counter. Each of these has a different combination and different dosages of vitamins and minerals. As a simple guideline, look at the label and choose a product that contains about one to two times the RDA or PDV for vitamins (RDA stands for "recommended daily allowance," while PDV stands for "percent daily value"). For instance, if the RDA for vitamin B_1 is 1.5 mg, a range of 1 to 3 mg should be adequate. The label will list percentages; for example, if the product contains 1.5 mg of B_1, the label will state that the dose is 100 percent of the RDA or PDV. If it contains 3 mg of B_1, the label will say 200 percent. As for the minerals, a lower percentage is adequate. Instead of one or two times the RDA, about half, or 50 percent, is all that would be necessary to take on a regular basis. Minerals have a tendency to accumulate in the body and lower amounts are needed. This is in contrast to most of vitamins, particularly the B-complex and C, which are easily flushed out of the system if larger-than-required doses are taken. You don't have to take these multivitamin and -mineral pills every single day. A few times a week would be fine.

If you don't consume fish on a regular basis, I recommend taking fish-oil capsules that supply 500 to 1000 mg of the important omega-3 fats EPA and DHA. As an alternative, you could take about a teaspoon of flaxseed oil each day, which also contains omega-3 oils (see Chapter 7 for details). These oils are important for proper brain function and vision. Another option is to take both the flax and the fish oil daily. One of my patients, James, is a twenty-eight-year-old strict vegetarian. As part of a mind-boosting program, I mentioned to him the importance of omega-3 fatty acids. He noticed an improvement in mood and alertness within two days of taking a tablespoon of flax oil daily. "I realized that I wasn't feeling that midafternoon slump and sleepiness anymore. Even my vision improved," he says. He is currently taking a teaspoon of flaxseed oil every day.

SUPPLEMENTS THAT IMPROVE MENTAL PERFORMANCE

There are times when the demands of our modern society may require that we perform at an extraordinary level. For instance, accountants during tax season often labor through fourteen-hour days. Lawyers must grind through long nights in order to prepare for a courtroom appearance. Hospital interns and residents are routinely asked to work twenty-four-hour or longer shifts, while remaining mentally alert and making life-and-death decisions. Writers, musicians, actors, and others in the arts may be required to create or perform for extended hours or during demanding situations. It is reassuring to know that there are natural supplements that one can rely on occasionally in order to enhance alertness, concentration, creativity, and mental capacity.

Having supervised many patients who regularly take mind sharpeners, I have observed that individual responses vary significantly. Although I provide a number for you to select from, the only way to find out for certain how you respond is to try these supplements yourself. As a rule, it is desirable for your initial doses to be low. You can always increase the dose if you do not notice an effect. I recommend that you have a thorough physical examination before trying new supplements and that a nutritionist or health-care practitioner adequately supervises you.

There is a large selection of mind-boosting supplements to choose from. The choice of a supplement would depend on a number of factors, including desired effect, cost, and individual preference. The effects of many supplements overlap. Most commonly you will notice an enhancement in alertness, focus, and motivation. Some supplements may also sharpen your vision, increase sex drive or sexual appreciation, or help you accomplish a particular project quicker and more efficiently.

The following is a list of natural supplements you can take *occasionally* to enhance your mental abilities. They are best taken in the morning or before lunch on an empty stomach, or with a small meal. As a general guideline, use these only a few days a month. If you take too high a dose, or a combination of two or more, you may feel overstimulated. For full details on how each one of these works, see the appropriate chapter in Part IV.

- A B-complex supplement supplying five to ten times the RDA can provide an elevation in mood and energy. As I mentioned earlier in this chapter, I recommend taking one to two times the RDA on a daily basis.
- Pantothenic acid is one of the B vitamins; at a dose of 250 to 500 mg, it enhances energy, alertness, and elevates mood.
- Coenzyme Q10 is an antioxidant that that also plays a role in the energy-production system in each cell. A dose of 30 to 90 mg in the morning leads to increased energy that is most often noticed by late afternoon or evening.
- Trimethylglycine, or TMG, is a lesser-known nutrient that has very noticeable effects on mood. Many people like the increase in energy and elevation of mood that come on a few hours after taking it. The usual dose is between 250 to 1000 mg. DMG, DMAE, and SAMe provide similar effects.
- Acetyl-L-carnitine, or ALC, is a nutrient involved in the energy-production system of cells. A dose of 250 to 750 mg improves energy, alertness, and mood within one to two hours.
- Tyrosine and phenylalanine are amino acids that convert into a brain chemical known as dopamine. A dose of 100 to 300 mg in the morning on an empty stomach leads to alertness within an hour. Some people take a small dose of these amino acids as a substitute for coffee. *High dosages can lead to overstimulation, racing of the heart, and irritability.*

- Once you have learned about the above nutrients, you can try others if you wish. These would include NADH, lipoic acid, vinpocetine, and pregnenolone. You can also learn about many of the energy-enhancing herbs such as ginseng, maca, gotu kola, and others, in Chapter 15.

As you can see, there are quite a number of options available. It may take trial and error to find the ideal nutrients that work well for your particular brain chemistry. It is likely that you will find positive effects not mentioned above. For instance, some of these nutrients may make you feel more talkative, clever, humorous, creative, or spontaneous. It's also possible, however, that too high a dose of some of these nutrients will interfere with your clarity of thinking or performance. It may take you several months to have a good understanding of how to best use these nutrients. Learning about mind boosters is a lifelong process. After years of research, I'm still constantly learning more myself. Again, it's important to emphasize that these nutrients should be used only occasionally, such as a few times a month.

MOOD-IMPROVING SUPPLEMENTS

Depression or low mood occurs commonly in the 25-to-40 age group, especially among women. A thorough medical evaluation is necessary before taking mood-elevating supplements. As a rule, a good diet, exercise, and other positive lifestyle habits can make an enormous difference. Supplements that work very well in improving mood are the B vitamins and the herb St. John's wort. Chapter 19 provides a complete step-by-step nutritional approach to treating depression.

In cases of premenstrual syndrome, therapies that may be helpful include B-complex vitamins, calcium at 1000 mg a day, pregnenolone at 5 to 10 mg in the morning, and 5-HTP or kava for anxiety. These supplements, except for the B-complex and calcium, are best reserved for the few days of the premenstrual stage. 5-HTP, or 5-hydroxytryptophan, is an amino acid–like nutrient that increases serotonin levels and works well for anxiety. A suggested dose is 25 mg on an empty stomach once or twice a day. Kava is an herb that effectively and safely reduces anxiety, and the suggested dose is 70 to 100 mg of the kavalactones (the active chemicals in kava) once or twice a day.

SUPPLEMENTS FOR STRESS

One potential problem that interferes with memory and clarity of thinking during one's twenties and thirties is stress, with severe cases leading to anxiety disorders. Herbal and nutritional supplements can address this problem.

Stress can occur on an occasional basis, or it can be ongoing. Kava, the antianxiety and antistress herb, can be very helpful when used occasionally. The usual dosage is 70 to 100 mg of the kavalactones (the active chemicals) once, twice, or three times a day. Kava helps in relaxation and does not significantly interfere with mental clarity. The best time to take it is in the late afternoon or early evening. Some find kava to be a good alternative to a martini.

5-hydroxytryptophan (5-HTP), the serotonin precursor, is another supplement that can be used occasionally to induce relaxation. The dosage is 25 to 50 mg on an empty stomach. The effects are often noticed within an hour. A high daytime dose, such as more than 50 mg, can cause sedation and the urge to sleep.

Additional herbs that can help as stress busters include ashwagandha, American ginseng, and reishi. The benefits from these herbs often become apparent after several days. If your diet is deficient in fish, supplements of fish oils or flaxseed oil could also help you with your adaptation to stressful situations.

STRATEGIES FOR SLEEP

Insomnia and restless nights are common in any age group. See Chapter 5 for specific step-by-step suggestions on how to improve your sleep quality. Melatonin, 5-HTP, and herbs such as ashwagandha and hops, can be used occasionally for a deeper sleep.

A NOTE TO VEGETARIANS

I supervise many patients who are vegetarian. When I inquire about their dietary intake, I find that a significant number have a tendency to overconsume carbohydrates at the expense of protein. Some do well on this nonmeat diet, but many find an improvement in their energy and mood when eating even small amounts of meat or dairy products. This may be due to an increased protein intake, or to the restoration of certain nutrients that are mostly found in meats, poultry, and fish. These nutrients include CoQ10, creatine, and carnitine. If you plan to remain a vegetarian, I recommend taking supplements of these nutrients. The daily dosage would be about 10 mg of CoQ10, 250 mg of carnitine, and 1 g of creatine.

Fish contains important omega-3 fats, such as EPA and DHA, that are necessary for brain health. If you are vegetarian or don't consume fish on a regular basis, supplementation with fish oils may be beneficial in terms of improved mood and clarity of thinking. A total of 500 to 1000 mg of DHA and EPA should be adequate. If you have an objection to taking fish-oil capsules, you could obtain omega-3 fats by consuming flaxseed oil, or take DHA capsules derived from algae.

PREGNANCY

Since most mind boosters have not been studied in pregnant women, no firm recommendations can be made. The addition of one to two times the RDA for vitamins is highly recommended, especially for folic acid. *A deficiency in folic acid can lead to neural-tube defects in the baby.*

Some women after delivery suffer from a condition called "postpartum depression," due to major changes in hormones, fatty acids, and neurotransmitters. See Chapter 19 on how to treat depression naturally. Fish oils may be helpful for this condition since these fatty acids are depleted in the mother due to the enormous quantities transferred to the fetus. Choline could also be helpful during or after pregnancy since a placental transport system removes choline from the mother in order to supply the phospholipid requirements of the fetus.

Summary

As a rule, most young, healthy individuals do not need to take any mind boosters on a regular basis as long as they have a good diet, sleep well, and follow proper lifestyle habits. The use of mind-boosting nutrients for special situations can help you be more alert, focused and productive.

SEVENTEEN

The Mind-Boosting Program for Ages 41 to 60

I hit age forty in November of 1997. I continue to be very productive and creative; however, if I don't take supplements, I feel less vital than I did a decade or two earlier. My energy level, memory ability, and libido are slightly lowered. I suspect that over the next two decades there may be a gradual decline in my cognitive abilities. I plan to try to slow this process by following the positive lifestyle habits I discuss in Part III, and also by taking some of the supplements mentioned in this book.

Men and women between the ages of 41 and 60 are often at their peak in terms of accomplishments and career advancement. Intellectual functioning during this time is still excellent, but subtle changes begin to become apparent. This is the time when hormone levels start declining. Both men and women often notice a dip in sexual drive, and perhaps a slight or moderate decrease in stamina. By late evening, some individuals feel drowsy and have difficulty staying alert past dinner.

Over the years, I have had many patients in this age group who, just like me, have benefited from the proper use of supplements. Gary, a fifty-one-year-old lawyer, had noticed a decline in alertness and focus for a number of years, along with occasional insomnia. He was not as productive at work as he had been in the past. Each afternoon he would find himself sleepy and tired, with the urge to take a nap. His sex drive had also been on a gradual decline. After a thorough medical history and examination, I started Gary on a simple dietary and supplement program that led to a tremendous improvement. Gary responded particularly well to a B-complex vitamin, fish oils, and ginkgo. Also, by substituting small frequent meals and snacks containing protein for a big carbohydrate lunch (he used to eat pasta regularly), he no longer had an afternoon slump. The twice-weekly use of small doses of nighttime melatonin improved his sleeping patterns. To help his sagging libido, I recommended the occasional use of DHEA during times when he wanted to be more sexually active. It worked.

Victoria, a fifty-four-year-old part-time interior designer, found her energy levels, mood, and cognitive abilities significantly improved with a combination of B vitamins, CoQ10, flaxseed oil, and ginseng. She was able to stay alert and focused all day, get household duties accomplished, and still have enough energy to enjoy her interior-design work twenty hours a week. "I have a renewed sense of well-being and joie de vivre," she says.

As you can see from the above two examples, the choice of supplements used by Gary and Victoria was different, but the end result—more energy and greater focus—was similar. There are many different mind-boosting options and combinations available.

The mind-boosting supplements and lifestyle habits that I recommend for this age group are similar to the ones I recommended for the 25-to-40 group, but more extensive. I separate these recommendations into three categories in order to accommodate individual preferences. I know some people who are reluctant to take many supplements, while others wish to take a dozen or more. If you are the former, the recommendations made in the "first-line" category should be sufficient for you. If you have an interest in taking more supplements, I have provided two additional categories. *Please consult a nutritionally oriented health-care provider before starting this mind-boosting program*. Make sure your provider is aware of the supplements you are taking, since some of them could potentially interfere with the medicines you may be prescribed. I recommend you read the top ten mind-boosting principles discussed in Chapter 2 before you start haphazardly swallowing pills.

FIRST-LINE SUPPLEMENTS FOR THE 41-TO-60 AGE GROUP

Begin with these simple suggestions:

- A multivitamin complex that contains one to three times the RDA or PDV is all that would be necessary to take on a regular basis. Your multimineral complex could include about 50 to 100 percent of the RDA for minerals. You don't have to take these multivitamin and -mineral pills every day; a few times a week would be fine. You might consider taking some of the B vitamins in their coenzyme form.
- In addition to the multivitamin pills, take additional antioxidants. I recommend vitamin C, between 100 and 250 mg, and vitamin E, between 20 and 100 i.u. You don't have to take these antioxidants every day.
- Make sure you have enough fish in your diet—or, if not, fish-oil supplements providing a total of 500 to 1000 mg of DHA and EPA would be adequate. If you're a strict vegetarian, take a half to one teaspoon of flaxseed oil a day to provide omega-3 oils.
- You can occasionally use an herbal adaptogen, such as ginseng, for additional mental and physical energy.

SECOND-LINE SUPPLEMENTS

If the supplements recommended above are not enough for you, consider adding one or more of the following under medical supervision.

Be careful when you start adding multiple supplements—their effects can be cumulative and overly energizing. In some cases the stimulation could cause you to feel irritable or anxious. Taking too many pills that have energizing properties, even if used in the morning, can cause insomnia. I recommend you learn the effects of each nutrient by itself before combining them. When you do combine, reduce the dosage of each.

Choose one of the following and learn its effects on your mind and body before trying another one:

- Ginkgo, at a dose of 40 mg, with breakfast or lunch, to improve memory and clarity of thinking. It may take several days before you notice the effects.
- CoQ10, at a dose of 10 to 30 mg, most mornings with breakfast, to increase energy levels.
- Pantothenic acid, at a dose of 100 mg, taken in the morning for enhanced energy and mood elevation.
- Trimethylglycine, or dimethylglycine, at a dose of about 100 mg, in the morning with or without food, to improve mood and energy.
- Acetyl-L-carnitine, at a dose of 250 mg, most mornings before or with breakfast, for enhanced alertness, clarity of thinking, and mood.

As much as possible, try to do some kind of physical activity during the day or evening that uses up the increased energy that the supplements provide. Even with all of these powerful nutrients, there's nothing like physical activity to make us feel good and give us a deep sleep at night.

THIRD-LINE SUPPLEMENTS

There are dozens of nutrients and herbs that have an effect on the mind. You will notice significant mental improvement from the suggestions provided in the first- and second-line therapies above. Most people will be quite content with these. However, it's possible that some of the above recommendations may not suit your needs, or that with time, you have an interest in trying additional supplements. Some users like to alternate between different nutrients. For these reasons I have provided additional options. *At this stage, it is very important that a health-care practitioner familiar with nutritional therapy closely supervise you.* If you add these nutrients, you will need to stop or reduce the dosage of the ones you are already on.

It's always preferable, if you are starting a new supplement, to do so during a period when you are not taking other supplements in order to determine its effects without interference. Try each nutrient on its own for at least a few days to learn about changes in alertness, mood, concentration, and potential side effects. If you plan to take these nutrients on a regular basis, I recommend using them only once or twice a week in order to avoid tolerance.

- Choline helps with focus and concentration. A dose of 250 mg is a good start. If you don't notice benefits from choline, try 100 to 250 mg of the activated form, sold as CDP-choline.
- Lipoic acid, 5 to 25 mg, can be taken most mornings with breakfast. Lipoic acid provides a subtle relaxation, and sharpness of vision. It is particularly helpful in regulating blood-sugar levels in diabetics.
- NADH at a dose of 2.5 or 5 mg once or twice a week in the morning, on an empty stomach, improves alertness, feelings of well-being, and libido.
- There are additional herbs and nutrients, such as vinpocetine, DMAE, and SAMe that you could explore with time. Please remember that the effects of many supplements are cumulative.

For instance, choline, CDP-choline, and DMAE all affect the acetylcholine system. Therefore, if you are combining them, you will need less of each. The effects of TMG, DMG, DMAE, and SAMe are also cumulative.

I do not recommend the amino acids phenylalanine and tyrosine in this age group since *high doses increase heart rate and may cause palpitations.*

Ask your physician if it would be appropriate to take a low dose of aspirin, such as a baby aspirin, or one-fourth of a 325 mg pill, a few times a week to thin the blood. This could improve circulation to the brain and reduce the risk for strokes or heart attacks.

HORMONE REPLACEMENT

It is a well-known fact that the production of many hormones declines with age. A phenomenon called *andropause* has been defined as the gradual decrease in men of the production of androgens such as the hormones DHEA and testosterone. This decline in hormone levels happens very gradually in men, in contrast to menopause in women where there is a sudden drop in estrogen levels as the ovaries stop producing estrogen. Although hormone replacement in women has been well researched, replacement in men is still a new concept and no definite answers are yet available.

In my judgment, there would be little need for hormone replacement in men younger than their mid-forties. Toward the late forties, you could consider starting certain hormones in minute doses if a health-care provider believes they would be beneficial. Hormones, especially DHEA and pregnenolone, are known to improve well-being and cognition, as well as increase sexual interest. Pregnenolone is a powerful memory booster. The question of estrogen and other hormone replacement in women continues to be a hotly debated issue. There are both benefits and risks from hormone replacement.

If hormone replacement is instituted, the dosages used should be very low. See Chapter 14 for full details on the benefits and risks of hormone replacement and recommendations for both men and women.

Cautions and Side Effects

Be very careful combining supplements if you have hypertension, heart disease, diabetes, thyroid problems, or other chronic medical conditions. Nutrients and hormones are powerful, and can interfere with medicines or alter the course of a medical condition, especially if you start taking many all at once.

Summary

Most individuals in the 41-to-60 age group do not suffer significant cognitive decline. However, there are a number of supplements that could offer benefits in improving alertness, motivation, productivity, sex drive, and clarity of thinking. If used properly, these supplements can also improve vision and mood, and help keep your mind youthful.

EIGHTEEN

The Mind-Boosting Program for Ages 61 and Over

With age, everyone experiences a decline in the ability to think, learn, and remember. In addition, there is a decline in sensory perception—vision is not as sharp and hearing deteriorates. Is this cognitive and perceptual decline inevitable, or are there steps we can take to slow this decline—or even reverse it? Fortunately, we now have easy access to dozens of nutrients that have a positive influence on brain function. The challenge is to find the right combination and the right dosage to provide the greatest benefit with the lowest risk.

The use of mind boosters in the 61-and-over age group is complicated by the fact that many seniors have preexisting medical conditions. Although some of the nutrients discussed in this book do not influence the course of a medical disease, others can have a significant effect. Therefore, I will discuss some of the common medical conditions in this age group and the best choice for supplements for each condition. This issue is further complicated by the fact that many older individuals are also taking pharmaceutical medicines to treat a particular condition. I'll discuss some of the potential interactions of drugs and nutrients, and even offer natural alternatives to some drugs.

The Encouraging Cases of Marge and Leonard

Marge is a seventy-one-year-old retired bookkeeper. "All my life I've worked with numbers," she said when she came to see me. "I used to have a great memory, but now I can't seem to remember simple things like phone numbers and where I put things. It's frustrating. I came home from shopping one afternoon and got the mail from the mailbox on the way into the house. There was a letter from my sister. I put the groceries in the kitchen and then I just couldn't remember where I put the letter. It took me twenty minutes, and I finally found it in the den."

Marge's case is typical of many whose memory falters with the aging process. After a thorough medical and neurological evaluation, I started her on a program that included a multivitamin, B-complex, and fish oils. She noticed slight benefits with these. Two weeks later, I added ginkgo, at a dose of 60 mg each morning. Marge found that ginkgo helped her to be more alert and focused. However, she wanted to take additional supplements. The next one I recommended was acetyl-L-carnitine. This nutrient proved to be extremely helpful. Marge noticed that her thinking was as clear as it had been a decade or two earlier. Her memory improved, and she was able to stay focused all day.

Leonard had a memory deficit similar to Marge's, but he also had noticed deterioration in his visual perception, energy levels, and libido. A complete medical evaluation did not reveal any conditions that accounted for his symptoms. Leonard was already taking a "one-a-day" multivitamin pill, with an additional 250 mg of vitamin C and 100 i.u. of vitamin E. My recommendations were to add a B-complex pill, a teaspoon of flaxseed oil daily (being a vegetarian, he did not want to take fish oils), 30 mg of CoQ10, and 60 mg of ginkgo. To help his sagging libido, I started Leonard on a combination of DHEA and pregnenolone, totaling 5 mg per day. Within two weeks, he noticed a marked improvement, and I recommended he reduce the frequency of the hormones' dosage to three times a week. His visual perception has now improved, most likely due to a combination of the vitamins, flaxseed oil, ginkgo, and pregnenolone. "Colors are sharper and clearer," he reports.

AGE-RELATED COGNITIVE DECLINE

In Chapter 1, I discussed the concept of normal brain aging; this natural decline in mental functioning is known as "*age-related cognitive decline*" (ARCD). This term is applied to persons generally fifty years and older who continue on a steady course of memory loss or decline in thinking ability. The deficits seen in ARCD are minimal compared to those seen in Alzheimer's disease, but they nevertheless can impair work productivity and interfere with quality of life. Listening to music, looking at art, traveling, and tasting food all become less enjoyable.

Several factors are involved in the gradual deterioration of mental capacities with age. Proper supplementation requires that we address most or all of these factors in order to slow down, stop, or even reverse several aspects of this mental decline. Following are specific recommendations on how to approach this decline from multiple directions.

TAKING CARE OF MEDICAL PROBLEMS

There are several medical problems that commonly occur in the 61-and-over age group. Many of these, or the medicines required to treat them, can accelerate cognitive decline. Have regular physical exams in order to make sure you don't have a treatable cause of mental impairment such as thyroid disease, depression, elevated blood sugar, or B_{12} deficiency. Eye and ear checkups are essential to find treatable causes such as glaucoma, cataracts, or impacted wax in the eardrums. When vision and hearing are impaired, the brain receives less stimulation. Proper glasses and hearing aids have a tonic effect on the brain. My father's mood and quality of life improved significantly after his eye doctor removed his cataracts and replaced them with new lenses. "I had forgotten how much pleasure is derived from seeing clearly," he tells me.

Let's discuss a few common medical conditions and see if there are alternative therapies that do not interfere with cognitive function.

Cardiovascular and cerebrovascular diseases—Elevated blood pressure can damage large and small blood vessels in the brain, and can lead to strokes. Strokes most commonly occur from a clot blocking blood flow to a specific part of the brain, or, less commonly, they can be a result of bleeding into the brain; the latter is called a brain hemorrhage. The use of aspirin and nutrients that have blood-thinning abilities can decrease the risk of a clot. However, caution is advised: Taking too many blood-thinning supplements in too-high doses can excessively interfere with coagulation, and increase the risk of bleeding (brain hemorrhage).

Blood pressure can often be controlled by antihypertensive drugs. A better option, though, is to reduce blood pressure through mild or moderate exercise, employ relaxation techniques, stop smoking, reduce body weight, incorporate fresh fruits and vegetables in your diet, and add magnesium, potassium, antioxidants, and omega-3 oils (flaxseed or fish oils). Preliminary research indicates that fish oils reduce the risk of heart-rhythm irregularities. Calcium channel blockers and beta-blockers are often used to control high blood pressure, but they are known to interfere with optimal mental functioning.

If you have hypertension or heart disease, good choices for mind boosters include omega-3 oils, ginkgo, choline, B vitamins, methyl donors, CoQ10, lipoic acid, and acetyl-L-carnitine. It is best you avoid the amino acids tyrosine and phenylalanine since they can increase blood pressure and cause heart-rhythm irregularities.

Elevated cholesterol—Many of the drugs (statins) used to decrease cholesterol and lipid levels in the blood can cause cognitive decline since they may also affect the production of cholesterol in the brain. Cholesterol is required for good brain-cell function, and is also needed to make steroid hormones such as pregnenolone, DHEA, estrogen, and testosterone. Overly low levels of cholesterol in the brain, as a consequence of drug use or excessive dietary restrictions, can lead to lowered mood and disturbances in the thinking process. If you have high cholesterol levels, many of the recommendations to lower blood pressure discussed above also apply to lowering cholesterol levels. In a study done at the University of California at Irvine, the addition of fish oils (1800 mg of EPA, 1200 mg of DHA) and garlic powder (1200 mg) for one month led to an 11 percent decrease in cholesterol levels and a 34 percent decrease in triglyceride levels (Morcos 1997). The effect of garlic supplements alone on cholesterol levels, however, is in dispute.

The mind boosters recommended above for those with heart disease would also apply to those with high cholesterol levels.

Osteoarthritis—Although nonsteroidal anti-inflammatory drugs (NSAIDs) such as ibuprofen can potentially help reduce the risk for Alzheimer's disease, they can also have significant side effects, including stomach ulcers, hearing loss, and kidney damage. A safer alternative for osteoarthritis would be to take 500 or 1000 mg of glucosamine three times a day. Glucosamine is a nutrient available over-the-counter. Chondroitin sulfate may also be helpful, at a dose of 400 mg three times a day. Vitamins C and D, omega-3 oils, and methyl donors are also potentially helpful.

Benign prostate hypertrophy—Known as BPH, prostate enlargement is not fatal but can cause a significant reduction in quality of life. The frequent nighttime awakenings to go to the bathroom interfere with the proper sleep necessary for full cognitive functioning. Doctors often prescribe the medicine finasteride (also known as Proscar) to block the conversion of testosterone to dihydrotestosterone (DHT), the hormone partly responsible for the growth of the prostate gland. However, finasteride may interfere with sexual drive and memory. You may wish to try the herbal extract saw palmetto, at a dose of 160 mg twice a day, which could potentially help you reduce your dose of finasteride. One advantage of finasteride, however, is that it can help preserve hair growth on the scalp.

Muscle wasting—As we age, we gradually lose our lean muscle mass. This decline can be partially reversed by the use of creatine. Creatine is a nutrient made of three amino acids. The use of 3 grams a day can help increase muscle size (see Chapter 20). Take a week off from creatine use each month, and a month off three times a year. Make sure your intake of protein is adequate since muscle tissue needs protein to maintain its mass.

Gastrointestinal problems—If you have a stomach ulcer or gastritis and take antacids and other medicines that reduce stomach acid, you could have problems absorbing some nutrients, particularly B_{12}; hence B_{12} shots could well provide you with great cognitive benefits.

Regulating Circadian Cycles

As we get older, there is an increase in the likelihood of disturbances in circadian rhythm. These rhythms affect various body functions, such as sleep cycles, body temperature, and hormone production. Exposure to sunlight or bright lights an hour or so a day can help assist in the regulation of these circadian cycles. As a rule, if you tend to feel sleepy before your normal bedtime, expose yourself to late-afternoon or early-evening sunlight. If you normally tend to be wired late at night, expose yourself to light in the morning. Light-exposure can be done simply by sitting near a window or taking a walk outside.

The occasional use of melatonin, in a dose of 0.3 to 1 mg once or twice a week, an hour or two before bed, can be used to help regulate your sleep cycle.

Supplements for ARCD

The deterioration of mental functioning with age is a consequence of numerous factors; these include decreased blood flow to the brain, inefficient energy production by the brain cells, changes in levels of brain chemicals and hormones, and deterioration of brain cells. Therefore, in order to keep the brain young, we need to slow down, stop, or even reverse as many of these processes as we can. I will first discuss how to deal with each of these processes, and then later I will give you a step-by-step guide to a mind-boosting nutritional program.

Improving bloodflow to the brain—Anything that helps slow the progression of atherosclerosis (hardening of the arteries) is beneficial to mental functioning. Atherosclerosis is often thought by the lay public to involve mostly the arteries of the heart—but hardening of the arteries with a reduction in blood flow can also occur commonly in the arteries supplying blood to the brain. Therefore, a diet emphasizing fresh vegetables and fruits, whole grains, proper antioxidant use, and a good intake of omega-3 oils can be helpful.

Ginkgo and omega-3 oils are a good choice for improving blood circulation since they have antiplatelet (or blood-thinning) activity. Aspirin is also a powerful antiplatelet agent. A small amount, such as a baby aspirin, or one-fourth of a 325 mg adult dose, taken a few times a week should be sufficient. Keep your dosages low when taking all three of them together.

Improving brain-cell energy metabolism—Brain cells need energy to function; they obtain most of this energy by metabolizing carbohydrates such as glucose. B vitamins are known to assist in this energy production. There are several additional nutrients that are involved in energy production within brain cells, including coenzyme Q10, acetyl-L-carnitine (ALC), and lipoic acid. In addition to their involvement in energy production, they also have good antioxidant properties. Many people notice cognitive improvements when supplementing with these mind energizers.

Studies have shown ALC to be beneficial in treating mild forms of cognitive decline. Arnold, a sixty-three-year-old engineer, says, "I take 250 mg of ALC on days when I need to keep focused. It helps me stay alert and helps me concentrate better. I think my work productivity has improved." CoQ10 also improves mental energy. Users find that they can think faster and stay more alert. A dose of 30 to 60 mg is generally adequate. Mary, a seventy-four-year-old patient with heart disease, finds that CoQ10 gives her more energy and improves her mood. Lipoic acid has not been tested in patients with ARCD, but small doses, such as 5 to 25 mg, sharpen vision and provide a relaxed sense of well-being.

Influencing neurotransmitter levels—Mood, behavior, memory, energy, and sex drive are influenced by brain chemicals, including serotonin, dopamine, norepinephrine, and acetylcholine. The levels of these brain chemicals can change with aging, and, fortunately, these levels can be manipulated with over-the-counter nutrients. For instance, choline and CDP-choline have an influence on acetylcholine; phenylalanine, tyrosine, and some of the B vitamins influence levels of dopamine and norepinephrine; and 5-HTP is a direct precursor to serotonin. The choice of nutrients depends on the specific condition being treated. For instance, Alzheimer's patients benefit from nutrients that influence acetylcholine levels, while patients with Parkinson's disease respond to nutrients that influence dopamine levels. Note that methyl donors increase the production of several neurotransmitters.

Influencing hormone levels—Similar to brain chemicals, over-the-counter hormones, such as DHEA and pregnenolone, influence mood, behavior, memory, energy, and sex drive. Hormones can be very beneficial, but misuse can lead to side effects.

Rebuilding brain cells—Our brains are made of billions of cells (neurons) that often deteriorate with age. Each neuron is enclosed by a lining called the "cell membrane." This membrane separates the insides of the cell from the outside. The cell membrane serves as a barrier, allowing certain necessary nutrients to come in, while restricting the entry of undesirable substances. This membrane consists mostly of different types of fats. Manipulation of the composition of these fats can significantly influence the function and efficiency of neurons. Several nutrients have the potential to do just this, including omega-3 oils and phospholipids.

Human research regarding the manipulation of brain-cell membranes with nutrients is still in its infancy. Therefore it is difficult to make firm recommendations regarding supplementation. Until we learn more, it may be appropriate to supplement with omega-3 oils and small amounts of phospholipids.

A STEP-BY-STEP GUIDE TO SUPPLEMENTS FOR THE 61-AND-OVER AGE GROUP

I separate the mind-boosting lifestyle habits and supplements that I recommend for the over-61 age group into three categories in order to accommodate individual preferences. Some people are reluctant to take many supplements, while others wish to take a dozen or more. If you are the former, the recommendations made in the "first-line" category should be sufficient for you. If you have an interest in taking more supplements, I have provided two additional categories. Please consult a nutritionally oriented health-care provider before starting this mind-boosting program. Make sure your provider is aware of the supplements you are taking since some of them could potentially interfere with the prescription medicines you may be taking. Before you take any supplements, review the top ten mind-boosting principles presented in Chapter 2.

Keep in mind that it's impossible to provide guidelines that would be appropriate to everyone reading this book. There are wide variations, at this stage in one's life, in state of health, mental function, absorption and metabolism of nutrients, and efficiency of the organs of metabolism and elimination, such as the liver and kidneys.

First-Line Therapy

I recommend a daily multivitamin complex that contains two to three times the recommended daily allowances (RDA) for the B vitamins. Your multimineral complex could include about 50 to 100 percent of the RDA for minerals. Some seniors might have difficulty absorbing vitamin B_{12} and may respond well to monthly injections.

- In addition to the multivitamin pills, take additional antioxidants; I recommend between 100 and 500 mg of vitamin C and between 30 and 200 i.u. of vitamin E.
- If you don't eat fish, fish-oil supplements providing a total of 500 to 1000 mg of the fatty acids EPA/DHA should be adequate. If you are a strict vegetarian, try a half to one teaspoon of flaxseed oil a day.
- Women may consider adding more soy products to their diet. Soy contains compounds that have estrogenic properties.

Second-Line Therapy

Most seniors will notice benefits from the first-line therapy suggested above. But if you feel you need more help, there are additional nutrients you can take. You don't have to take all of these supplements all of the time. If you are financially limited, or don't like popping too many pills, take only a couple of supplements a day. If you are interested in trying many supplements, start with one or two, and gradually add more. Remember that the effects of these nutrients are *cumulative.* If you're not careful, you could get overstimulated and experience insomnia, which would be counterproductive to good health. As you add more supplements, reduce the dosage of the ones you already take. Ideally, I recommend you learn the effects of each nutrient by itself before combining them.

- To improve blood flow to the brain, take 40 mg of ginkgo with breakfast or lunch. Energy metabolism can be improved by taking 100 to 250 mg of acetyl-L-carnitine, 10 to 30 mg of CoQ10, or 5 to 25 mg of lipoic acid. Hormone replacement with DHEA or pregnenolone can potentially benefit bone formation, mood, libido, memory, and overall cognitive function. Pregnenolone can, in some individuals, improve hearing and vision; but there are potential side effects to hormone replacement if misused. See Chapter 14 for full details and dosage guidelines.
- Melatonin can be used at a dose of 0.3 to 1 mg one or three times a week, an hour or two before bed, to improve sleep.

Third-Line Therapy

There are dozens of nutrients and herbs that have an effect on the mind. You will notice significant improvements from the suggestions provided in the first- and second-line therapies. The majority of individuals will be quite content with these. However, I know individuals who are very curious to learn more about supplements. I have provided additional options for those with this inclination.

It's always best to start a new supplement when you are not taking other supplements; that way you can determine its effects without interference. Try each nutrient on its own for at least a few days to learn about changes in alertness, mood, concentration, and potential side effects. If you plan to take the following nutrients on a regular basis, I recommend using them only once or twice a week to avoid tolerance.

- Choline helps with focus and concentration; a dose of 250 mg is a good start. If you don't notice benefits from choline, try 100 to 250 mg of the activated form, sold as CDP-choline. TMG, and its cousin DMG, at a dose of 100 mg, provide an improvement in alertness and mood. NADH, at a dose of 2.5 or 5 mg, improves mood, alertness, and perhaps even sex drive. Limit the use of NADH to once or twice a week since tolerance to this nutrient can develop quickly. NADH is best taken in the morning on an empty stomach.

- There are additional nutrients, herbs, and herbal extracts—such as DMAE, SAMe, ginseng, maca, and vinpocetine—that you could explore with time. Whether supplements of PS and lecithin improve cognitive abilities in the aged has yet to be determined.

Cautions and Side Effects

Ginkgo biloba, feverfew, garlic, ginger, vinpocetine, aspirin, and high doses of vitamin E may increase the risk of bleeding in patients taking antithrombotic (blood-thinning) agents.

Always take low dosages when you combine multiple supplements. This may require that you break a tablet into small portions, or open a capsule to take a fraction of the contents.

Summary

Although our bodies and brains are preprogrammed to aging, there are several steps we can take to slow this process. Many of the supplements I discuss in this book can have an enormous benefit in improving memory, vision, clarity of thinking, motivation, joie de vivre, and creativity. Let's be appreciative that these nutrients are readily available.

PART VI

Natural Prescriptions for Depression, Vision Enhancement, Alzheimer's, and Parkinson's Disease

NINETEEN

Supplements That Fight Depression

A happy, healthy mind can be compared to a pond with a high water level. There may be many rocks of all sizes and shapes at the bottom of the pond, but these rocks are not visible and they do not interfere with the pond's serenity and tranquility. The rocks at the bottom represent all the minor and major traumas that we have been exposed to, or are currently experiencing, as part of living on this sometimes hostile and unforgiving planet. They represent embarrassments, emotional breakups, childhood traumas, past and current illnesses, pain, and all the other hurts that are the inevitable rites of passage that all of us go through on our way to adulthood. Yet a pond with a high water level covers up these rocks: they are no longer visible and no longer interfere with the surface tranquility.

Now imagine the water level of this pond gradually depleting. Little by little, as the water level lowers, the tips of the larger rocks begin to show. As the water level drops even farther, medium-sized and even smaller rocks become apparent.

I sometimes recount this analogy to those with low mood or clinical depression. I mention that, even though it's very important to try to resolve as many past and current issues and hurts (the rocks) as possible through self-analysis, behavioral therapy, psychotherapy, and other methods, it's just as important to bring the level of the water back up. The level of the water (i.e., brain chemicals) can often successfully be raised by nutritional therapies. Once you restore the proper amounts and balance of your brain chemicals, and provide the nutritional support for your brain cells to work more efficiently, many of the frustrations and hurts that you have experienced in the past, or are currently experiencing, won't seem nearly as challenging or disturbing.

NUTRIENTS TO THE RESCUE

How good we feel is largely dependent on the levels and interactions of a number of neurotransmitters in the brain, including serotonin, norepinephrine, and dopamine. Low mood or clinical depression is mostly due to an imbalance or shortage of some of these neurotransmitters at important sites in the central nervous system. However, disturbances in mood can also result from medical diseases, nutrient deficiencies, improper fatty-acid intake, and inefficient energy production within cells.

Antidepressants were first introduced back in the 1950s. Since then, a number of different classes of antidepressants have been created. Many of these medicines have benefited countless patients by relieving their symptoms of despair. But there are nutritional factors that could be just as effective as drugs.

With the current availability of a number of natural supplements that influence mood, it is now possible, in my opinion, to not rely on pharmaceutical medicines for the therapy of mild—and probably moderate—depression. Perhaps even some cases of severe depression could respond, at least partially, to a suitable combination of natural nutrients and herbs. Supplements can also be used in conjunction with behavioral and cognitive therapies, and even in combination with lower dosages of pharmaceutical antidepressants. Traditional psychiatrists are beginning to incorporate natural therapies in their practice;

one of the first mood-influencing herbs to gain wide respect among medical doctors was St. John's wort.

There are different types of depression, and each person has a unique biochemistry. Some cases of depression are due to low levels of serotonin, while other cases are due to low levels of dopamine or norepinephrine. Still others may be due to abnormalities in the energy production of brain cells, abnormal cell membranes, or nerve damage. It is unlikely that a single therapy will provide complete relief to patients who are clinically depressed.

Please keep in mind that the suggestions discussed in this chapter are only guidelines. I recommend that you supplement with these natural nutrients only under the close supervision of a health-care practitioner. He or she should make sure you do not have any obvious medical conditions that could account for your depression, such as thyroid disease, tumors, or anemia.

First-Line Therapy

The health of the body is intricately involved with the health of the brain. I highly recommend you review the suggestions in Part III regarding diet, stress reduction, good sleep, and physical activity. These alone can often be curative. Many cases of depression may also be due to feeling alone and unloved. Try to find a community of caring individuals, where you feel part of a group. Pets are also wonderful companions. Relying exclusively on supplements to elevate mood, without making the effort to improve lifestyle habits or to develop loving connections, will not provide you with full relief.

Follow these step-by-step guidelines:

- Eat small, frequent meals throughout the day that consist of a well-proportioned balance between protein, fat, and complex carbohydrates. I find vegetarians sometimes suffer from low mood because they consume excess carbohydrates at the expense of adequate protein and the right kinds of fats. A large intake of carbohydrates can make one sluggish and sleepy.

- Take a multivitamin pill each morning that supplies about 100 percent of the RDA or PDV for most vitamins. In addition, take a B-complex pill supplying five to ten times the RDA for the B vitamins. You might also consider the coenzyme forms of the B vitamins, especially if you are older or you do not respond to the regular B vitamins. After a month of taking five to ten times the RDA for the B vitamins, reduce your daily intake to two to three times.
- Take a combination of a few antioxidants in small doses, including 30 to 100 units of vitamin E and 100 to 250 mg of vitamin C.
- A multimineral pill that includes about 50 to 100 percent of the RDA for minerals is recommended.
- Take fish-oil capsules with meals, totaling about 2 to 4 grams a day of the omega-3 fatty acids EPA and DHA. After the first month, reduce the dosage to 1 to 2 grams a day. Strict vegetarians can instead take a teaspoon of flaxseed oil.

Desiree, a thirty-eight-year-old homemaker with mild depression, is a typical example of a person who responded quite well to the above nutrient supplementation. "I noticed the most dramatic effects from the B vitamins," she says, "although the addition of the flaxseed oil improved my alertness, too. I can now function all day without being tired, and my husband mentioned that I was acting more cheerful."

Second-Line Therapy

If, after adopting the above regimen for two weeks, your depression has not been adequately treated, you can now add more nutrients.

Take a St. John's wort pill with breakfast, at a dose of 300 mg, standardized to 0.3 percent hypericin content. This herb has a wonderful ability to improve one's outlook on life.

If after a few days you don't notice any benefits, you can add a second St. John's wort pill either with breakfast or with lunch. Although most studies involving this herb have been done using three pills a day, I recommend the lower dosage. I have found that the risk for side effects such as insomnia increases when the dosage is increased to three pills a day. Instead of the third pill, it may be preferable to rely on different mood-elevating nutrients.

Michael, a forty-two-year-old systems engineer, suffered from a moderate case of depression following a divorce. The effects of St. John's wort were dramatic. "Within three days after starting the St. John's wort, I definitely noticed an uplifting of mood. It seemed like my emotional pain was not as intense." Michael stayed on St. John's wort for a period of four months, and successfully came off the herb without any further depression.

Third-Line Therapy

Let's assume you've tried the above therapies for four weeks, but you still need help. Here are additional suggestions:

- Start with tyrosine, at a dose of 100 mg, in the morning on an empty stomach. This amino acid is particularly helpful if you have difficulty staying alert. Many people find it to be a good substitute for caffeine. Tyrosine is more suitable for those younger than forty-five, since older individuals, and those with heart problems, can develop heart palpitations with high dosages. If you're taking St. John's wort, do not take high doses of tyrosine; the effects are potentially cumulative.
- After a week, add a dose of 30 mg of CoQ10 in the morning. This nutrient can increase energy levels and is particularly helpful for those who have low energy associated with their depression.
- Additional nutrients that can be added over the next few weeks include TMG, DMG, SAMe, or pantothenic acid at a dose of 100 to 250 mg, in the morning. All of these nutrients have excellent mood- and energy-elevating properties. Carnitine at 250 mg a day is another nutrient that increases energy levels.

Daisy, a twenty-eight-year-old clothing-store manager, could not tolerate St. John's wort, due to an allergic reaction, but found the combination dosage of 100 mg tyrosine, 30 mg CoQ10, and 100 mg pantothenic acid was extremely helpful in "beating the blahs," as she called it. Her low mood was a consequence of a relationship breakup. She stayed on these nutrients for three months, after which she gradually eliminated the tyrosine. She now occasionally takes only the pantothenic acid and the CoQ10, along with some of the nutrients mentioned in the first-line therapy.

Fourth-Line Therapy

Thus far, you have been presented with quite a few options. Chances are your symptoms may have already responded adequately to the above regimen. However, if your depression has not improved significantly, it's time to try additional supplements. *At this stage you must be very carefully and closely supervised by your health-care provider because the risk of interactions between the nutrients can increase significantly.* There is also a possibility of overstimulation when too many energizers are used. Some of these nutrients can slowly accumulate in the system, and you may find you need lower dosages with time. The treatment of depression is a dynamic process, and dosages of nutrients and medicines have to be adjusted up or down on a regular basis. If your depression lifts, don't continue to add more nutrients; instead try to minimize the dosages and the number of nutrients you are taking.

- There are quite a number of other options available. For instance, the herb ginseng can provide a sense of vitality and well-being. If your depression is associated with anxiety, the serotonin precursor 5-HTP can be helpful. The nighttime dosage is 25 to 50 mg, about an hour or two before bed, on an empty stomach, while the daytime dosage is 25 mg, anytime during the day. Taking 5-HTP at night will help you get a deeper sleep. At most, 5-HTP should be used only four days a week, and for no longer than two months continuously. After a month's break, you can resume taking 5-HTP again. You can cycle 5-HTP two months on and one month off, if needed.

- For a deeper sleep, try the occasional use of melatonin, at a dose of 0.3 to 0.5 mg once or twice a week, an hour or two before bed on an empty stomach. High doses of melatonin, such as more than 2 mg, when used nightly, can lower mood in some individuals. Since 5-HTP and melatonin work in similar ways to induce sleep, the dosages of each need to be reduced if you're planning to take them together.
- Two additional supplements to consider are NADH and acetyl-L-carnitine. NADH can be taken at a dose of 2.5 or 5 mg two or three times a week, in the morning on an empty stomach. NADH improves mood, energy, and sex drive. Since it is a relatively new nutrient, I recommend using it, at most, only three times a week until more research is available. Acetyl-L-carnitine has mood-elevating properties, and 100 to 250 mg is a good starting dose. As with most stimulants, it is best taken before breakfast or lunch.
- Older people, especially those with a sluggish libido, may find the addition of hormones, in conjunction with the nutrients, to be extremely helpful. DHEA or pregnenolone, or a combination of the two, can be started at a dose of 5 mg. For long-term use, I do not recommend exceeding a dose of 2 to 5 mg a day. Take a break of at least a week from the use of these hormones each month.

Summary

Combining supplements in the therapy of depression is a relatively new concept for most doctors trained in traditional medicine. Even doctors who practice complementary medicine are still in the early stages of learning the appropriate amounts to combine these nutrients. Due to the shortage of published information in this area, it is very important that the mixing of supplements be done in a cautious way—always starting with low dosages.

The intelligent combination of natural vitamins, nutrients, herbs, and hormones can have powerful mood-elevating effects. At the very least, the use of nutrients could allow for a reduction in the dosages of pharmaceutical antidepressants.

TWENTY

Supplements That Sharpen Vision and Hearing

Do you remember how crisp, sharp, and beautiful scenery looked years ago? Do you recall sitting for hours in your bedroom playing records or CDs over and over again, appreciating the melodies, rhythms, and the musical contribution of each instrument? Do you now find that some of the enchantment from looking and listening has faded away?

As we age, we lose some of our perceptive abilities. This is due in part to degeneration of nerve cells in the eyes and ears. Music and other sounds are no longer as delightful as in our teenage years; going to a concert does not seem as exciting. A castle in Europe, a swan floating on a still pond, a delicate daisy, or rugged mountain scenery may not impress us as much. We lose our ability to notice fine details and to differentiate subtle shades of colors. Has this enchantment disappeared forever, or are there ways to return the visual and auditory magic that life offers?

I am glad to report that the proper use of many of the nutrients discussed in this book can help restore, at least partially, the magic of seeing and hearing that you may have long forgotten exists. Most of this chapter will deal with visual enhancement—there is more information on how to improve vision with natural supplements than on how to improve hearing.

I will first review two important parts of the eye, the lens and the retina; then I will discuss nutrients that enhance vision and hearing.

The Lens

The lens and the retina are the two crucial parts of the eye involved in visual acuity. The *lens* is a disk-shaped transparent structure, about half the size of a M&M candy, that helps focus light on the retina, an area in the back of the eye. Excessive sunlight exposure, high blood-sugar levels (particularly in diabetics), smoking, and a shortage of antioxidants can cause damage to the lens, leading to dark areas. With time, these dark areas grow and become more prevalent, leading to the development of cataracts. When looking into the eye with a special flashlight called an ophthalmoscope, a cataract appears brownish or black. These dark areas interfere with vision because they block light from reaching the retina. Little can be done nutritionally to correct a cataract once it has formed, but a cataract can be removed surgically and replaced with an artificial lens.

The Retina

The retina lies in the back of the eye and is composed of cells called rods and cones. The retina gathers light and visual information from the outside world. This information is then transmitted through a special nerve bundle, called the optic tract, to an area in the back of the brain called the visual cortex. The visual cortex, in turn, interprets this information. Thus, vision can be improved at the retinal level, or at the level of transmission and interpretation of this optical information.

There's a small area in the retina called the *macula*, where vision is at its sharpest. Millions of elderly people suffer from macular degeneration, the leading cause of blindness in people over the age of fifty. Macular degeneration causes a gradual loss of vision and eventual blindness, and is caused at least partly by oxidation. Hence antioxidants are helpful in keeping both the lens and the retina healthy.

PROTECTING YOUR EYES

The lens, retina, macula, and other parts of the eye can be protected with the proper intake of antioxidants. Almost all the antioxidants are likely to have a positive influence on eye health. Of particular importance are vitamins C and E, selenium, and the carotenoids found in fruits and vegetables. Two particular carotenoids, called lutein and zeazanthin, play an important role in protecting eye tissue in the macula from damage by free radicals. Corn, eggs, green leafy vegetables, peppers, red grapes, and pumpkins are some of the foods rich in lutein and zeazanthin. You can also find carotenoids and flavonoids in many herbs, including milk thistle and bilberry.

For optimal vision protection, I recommend you include a variety of whole foods in your diet and take antioxidants. At this point, we don't know exactly what amounts and combinations of antioxidants will ensure optimal protection. You may wish to follow some of the suggestions provided in Chapter 11.

NUTRIENTS THAT SHARPEN VISION

Good eyesight requires more than just eating carrots. Most everything that you do to improve your overall health will, in the long run, influence the health of your eyes.

After years of supervising patients who take mind boosters, and trying various supplements myself, I am now aware of many that have an immediate effect on visual perception. Unfortunately, very little information has been published regarding the influence of different nutrients on the visual system. Hence, much of the information in this chapter is anecdotal, based on my professional and personal experiences.

Following is a list of supplements that improve eyesight. You are likely to notice the effects the very day you take them, and sometimes even within an hour or two. Generally, the higher the dose, the more obvious the visual improvement; however, the risk of side effects also increases as the dosage is increased. The combination of two or more nutrients often has a synergistic effect.

The mechanisms of action of these supplements can involve several pathways, such as raising levels of brain chemicals, improving blood circulation to the eye, or altering the fatty-acid composition of rods and cones and brain cells. I often find that visual changes are not as apparent when one is in broad sunlight. Going indoors—for instance, into a shopping mall—can help one become more aware of the visual enhancement. Late afternoon, early evening, and cloudy days are also good times to notice the visual changes.

Omega-3 oils—Just like the rest of the cells in the brain, the cells of the retina—the rods and the cones—contain long-chain fatty acids. The most prominent of these fatty acids in the eye is an omega-3 fatty acid called DHA. In my experience, I have found that the omega-3 oils, generally found in fish and flaxseed, enhance visual perception. I notice improved color perception and depth of vision, enhanced night and distance vision, and overall enhancement in visual awareness after several days of taking flaxseed oil or fish-oil capsules. In order to notice quicker results—i.e, within two or three days—the dosages need to be significant. For instance, most people need to take several grams of a combination EPA/DHA fish-oil supplement or a table-spoon or two of flaxseed oil. Once you notice an improvement, you can reduce your dosage of fish oils to one or two grams a day, or a teaspoon of flaxseed oil.

Burton J. Litman, Ph.D., at the National Institutes of Health in Rockville, Maryland, is an expert in the biochemistry of vision. He says,

> Each rod contains thousands and thousands of DHA molecules stacked up on each other. DHA is necessary for rhodopsin to function. [Rhodopsin is a protein in retinal rod cells that helps with perception of light.] Each day a small percentage of the

> DHA is taken away and replaced by new DHA. Dietary intake of fish oils [or omega-3 oils] could have an influence on these rods. As we age, we lose some of the phospholipids in brain-cell membranes that contain DHA and these are replaced by saturated lipids.

Since we lose some of the DHA present in the retina with age, it's quite possible that someday we may discover that dietary replacement of the proper fatty acids, especially in the elderly, will improve visual, and perhaps auditory perception. I personally notice an enhancement in visual perception when I supplement with several grams of fish oils. Sometimes it takes me a few days of taking high doses of fish oils to notice a difference, although I have noticed an effect the first day if I take several grams.

Pregnenolone is an interesting hormone that not only improves vision, but also enhances awareness. By this, I mean you become more aware of your environment; scenery, works of art, patterns on clothing, plants, and architecture that you might normally overlook suddenly become eye-catching. I notice the effects within a few hours of taking a dose of 10 or 20 mg. However, it takes several days of supplementing with pregnenolone at a smaller dosage to notice the visual effects. Colors become brighter and clearer, and shapes and patterns are more obvious. Reports from patients indicate that about a third notice these dramatic effects. Barbara, a television producer from Orange County, California, relates an interesting response:

> I took 10 mg of pregnenolone in the morning for three days and didn't feel much. On the fourth day, while waiting at a traffic light, I noticed how beautiful the red color looked. The light turned green and I kept looking at it in amazement. I had never seen a traffic light look so beautiful. I had to move soon, though, because cars behind me started honking. I arrived at the shop-

ping mall and now realized the beauty of the planted flowers. I kept staring at them for a long time.

Ted, a physician from San Diego, says, "I had stopped at a gas station to fill up the tank when I noticed an American flag by the pump. I had never seen red and blue colors that intense. It came to mind that I had taken pregnenolone for the first time that morning, at a dose of 20 mg. I will always remember that flag at the gas station."

The improved visual appreciation can lead some individuals to a dramatic appreciation of art. But don't take a high dose of pregnenolone and visit an art gallery or antique store while carrying a credit card. I did once and ended up purchasing antiques on the spur of the moment, a few more than I really needed—they looked so beautiful!

The visual effects from pregnenolone can last from a few hours, to all day. Unfortunately, pregnenolone has a downside. High doses can lead to side effects, including overstimulation, irritability, headaches, and acne—and *very* high doses, such as 30 mg or more, can cause heart palpitations in individuals prone to heart irregularities; sensitive individuals may notice skipped beats on a dose as low as 10 mg. Until more is known about pregnenolone's long-term health effects, I recommend its use for hormone-replacement therapy only in low dosages, such as 1 to 5 mg; 10 or 20 mg can be taken occasionally, such as once or twice a month, by healthy individuals who have no major medical problems. If you don't notice an effect from taking the oral pills, try the sublingual (under-the-tongue) form.

Pantothenic acid is one of the B vitamins (B_5). A dose of 100 to 500 mg taken in the morning improves clarity of vision, usually noticeable in the late afternoon, and continuing until bedtime. As with many nutrients that cause alertness, high dosages, even when taken in the morning, can interfere with nighttime sleep. Pantethene, the coenzyme form of pantothenic acid, produces similar visual improvement on a much lower dose of 25 to 50 mg.

NADH—In August of 1998, I took a trip to Alaska. During my three-week sojourn in this beautiful state, I had the opportunity to try some of the nutrients I had brought along. On my second day of the trip, I was in a van with a group driving down from Anchorage to Homer. All around me were majestic snowcapped peaks and lush, green meadows dotted with spruce trees. The day was overcast and windy as we pulled up to a scenic point. The wind was creating small ripples over the dark blue waters of the Cook Inlet. I had taken 5 mg of NADH, the coenzyme form of the B-vitamin niacin, before breakfast, and now, two hours later, the effects were becoming apparent. Not only did I have a pleasant sense of well-being, but, also, the beauty of this Alaskan scenery was coming to life. I realized at that moment how fortunate we are to have access to many natural supplements that not only improve health, but also enhance our appreciation of life and the natural beauty of this planet. I became even more encouraged to continue my quest to learn as much as I could about nutrients that improve quality of life and to share this knowledge with the public.

I'm not sure exactly how NADH enhances vision. It likely has to do with raising levels of the brain chemical dopamine since, in my experience, dopamine-enhancing nutrients and medicines improve visual perception. Any supplement or drug that enhances dopamine levels can improve vision, at least temporarily.

Phenylalanine, tyrosine, and **acetyl-tyrosine** convert into dopamine. Improvement in visual clarity is generally noticed within hours after taking a dose of 100 to 500 mg. Be aware, however, that high dosages induce irritability and anxiety.

Acetyl-L-carnitine is an antioxidant involved in energy utilization within cells. A dose of 500 mg in the morning before breakfast works within two to three hours to induce a pleasant visual and mental clarity.

CDP-choline enhances acetylcholine production, but may also influence dopamine levels. Visual clarity is apparent within a few hours after taking 250 or 500 mg.

TMG, **DMG**, **DMAE**, and **SAMe** are methyl donors that have similar effects of sharpening vision, most likely due to an increase in levels of brain chemicals. DMG is available in sublingual form and the visual effects are apparent within an hour of melting a pill under the tongue.

Lipoic acid is an antioxidant that enhances glucose use in brain and eye cells. Usually a dose of 25 to 50 mg improves visual clarity. The effects are noticeable by late afternoon or evening.

Vinpocetine is an herbal extract that improves blood circulation to the brain. A dose of 10 to 20 mg leads to visual clarity within one or two hours.

There are many other supplements that improve visual appreciation, but their effects are subtle. These nutrients and herbs include the *B vitamins, CoQ10, 5-HTP, ginkgo, kava, St. John's wort, and some of the adaptogenic herbs, such as ginseng.* Lecithin, phosphatidylserine, creatine, and antioxidant vitamins such as C and E do not have an immediate effect on visual perception.

AUDITORY ENHANCERS

Formal research regarding the field of hearing improvement from the use of supplements is practically nonexistent, and my experience with nutrients that improve hearing is limited compared to my experience with those supplements that improve vision. My eyesight is normally 20/30, with a slight astigmatism; hence, I can appreciate even subtle changes in vision that some nutrients provide. Nevertheless, my hearing is excellent, and it is difficult for me to notice subtle improvements. Nevertheless, there are certain nutrients that I am quite certain have a definite influence on hearing; these include pregnenolone, NADH, and pantothenic acid.

I first became aware of pregnenolone's effect on auditory appreciation while driving back to Los Angeles from a medical conference in Palm Springs, California. It was early evening, and I was changing the stations on the car radio when I realized that just about every song was pleasant to my ear, whether it was classical, jazz, rock, Celtic, or country. That morning I had taken 20 mg of the hormone. I hadn't enjoyed listening to music that much since my teenage years. I have since noticed this auditory enhancement on multiple occasions.

The first time I noticed the effects of NADH on hearing was while dining at a Peruvian restaurant. They were playing Andean flute music in the background at a very low volume. I sat there mesmerized, in full appreciation of the gentle flute notes, while my three friends at the table could hardly hear, let alone appreciate, the melody. My dose that morning was 5 mg.

Additional nutrients that can potentially enhance auditory appreciation include pantothenic acid, the amino acids phenylalanine and tyrosine, the methyl donors, and some of the adaptogenic herbs such as ginseng. I am quite certain we will eventually discover many other supplements that improve hearing.

Summary

The use of supplements to improve vision and hearing is a relatively new concept in medicine. We are living in exciting times; it has only been in the last few years that we have had so many nutritional options available to us. It's comforting to know that we don't have to succumb to the ravages of time. We can see more sharply and hear more clearly by intelligently using nutrients and herbs.

However, I must add that not everyone notices visual effects from taking nutrients. The young who already have excellent vision may not notice the subtle improvements that occur. The elderly, particularly those who have advanced cataracts or damaged retinas, also may not respond. People also differ depending upon how in tune they are with their senses. Some individuals can perceive very subtle changes, while others require massive dosages before they realize something different is happening. I have one thirty-year-old male patient who hardly ever notices any effects from supplements no matter what he takes. Another patient, a forty-four-year-old woman, has excellent perception skills. For instance, she will notice a visual effect from 2 mg of pregnenolone. I, too, am very sensitive to subtle changes. Over my many years of taking different supplements in varying dosages, I have developed the skill of observing minute changes that occur in mood, energy, alertness, and vision. This quality has helped in my evaluation of nutrients.

TWENTY-ONE

Supplements for Patients with Alzheimer's Disease

Alzheimer's disease (AD), a progressive deterioration in mental functioning first described by Alois Alzheimer in 1907, affects more than 4 million Americans. Onset most commonly occurs in one's eighties, although it has been known to start as early as age thirty. One of the major cognitive problems with AD is the inability to acquire new knowledge. Loss of the sense of smell is common, and the mental deterioration proceeds to affect language and motor skills.

With the continued aging of the population, the prevalence of AD is expected to rise over the next few decades. One of the reasons medical therapies for this condition have generally been unsuccessful is that doctors have focused on a "one pill" approach. Unlike Parkinson's disease, which is due to damage to a small, specific area in the brain, it has been difficult to identify a precise area in the brain associated exclusively with AD. But growing evidence suggests that the memory and learning deficits associated with AD are due to the degeneration of brain cells that rely on the brain chemical acetylcholine.

Several theories have been advanced in the past few decades regarding the causes of AD. These include genetics, toxic-metal excess, damage to brain cells by oxidation, infections, nutritional deficiencies, dysfunction of the blood-brain barrier, and side effects of medicines.

TREATMENT STRATEGIES FOR ALZHEIMER'S DISEASE

While scientists have not fully determined the actual causes of Alzheimer's disease, a number of treatment options have been proposed or tried over the years; these include the following:

- Exposure to sunlight, and sleep-pattern restoration.
- Therapy with B vitamins, and lowering homocysteine levels.
- The use of antioxidants.
- Providing acetylcholine precursors.
- Enhancing cellular energy with CoQ10 and acetyl-L-carnitine.
- Hormone therapies with estrogen, testosterone, and DHEA.
- Providing anti-inflammatory agents such as aspirin or ibuprofen.
- Blocking the breakdown of acetylcholine with pharmaceutical drugs.
- Improving blood flow to brain cells.
- Mood improvement through nutrients and herbs.

Following, I'll examine the potential benefit of each of the above approaches. Later in the chapter I provide step-by-step guidelines on how to best combine nutrients. Please keep in mind that no studies have been done on the combination of nutrients that I plan to discuss. Studies using combination therapies are rarely undertaken; hence, we would have to wait a very long time to have scientists formally evaluate this approach. There are currently no effective pharmaceutical drugs for treating AD. If someone you know has AD, I believe it is worthwhile exploring nutritional therapies even though the necessary studies are not available. One can always resort to pharmaceutical medicines if this nutritional approach is not helpful.

A rational plan, then, is to follow a multipronged and comprehensive approach in targeting the different types of problems that contribute to mental decline. This approach could perhaps stop, or at least delay, the relentless degeneration that occurs in AD. It is my hope that some individuals are even able to reverse their cognitive decline through this comprehensive approach.

Light Therapy

People afflicted with Alzheimer's often suffer disturbances in circadian rhythm, which affects body functions such as sleep cycles, temperature, alertness, and hormone production. Exposure to sunlight or bright lights, half an hour to an hour a day, could help correct the sleep disturbance and assist in the regulation of the circadian cycles. This light exposure can be attained simply by sitting near a window or taking a walk outdoors. The occasional use of melatonin at night, in a dose of 0.3 to 1 mg, one or two hours before bed, can help reset the circadian rhythm and ensure a deeper sleep. Patients with AD produce much less melatonin than in other individuals of the same age (Liu 1999).

Vitamin-B Therapy

Several studies have indicated that patients with AD have deficiencies in some of the B vitamins (McCaddon 1994). Costing only pennies a day, the administration of a multivitamin supplement, containing a few times the recommended daily allowance for the B vitamins, is a cost-effective and safe first step in the therapy of AD.

All of the Bs are important since they each work in multiple ways to improve brain function. Further, B_6, folic acid, and B_{12} are helpful in reducing levels of homocysteine. A study of hundreds of British patients has revealed a link between Alzheimer's and high levels of homocysteine (Refsum 1998). "It is a very promising finding," says Professor Helga Refsum of Norway's Bergen University. Refsum, like many scientists, is cautious about recommending supplements, stressing that so far the results have only revealed an association, not a direct cause and effect. She tells me, "We, as physicians, should refrain from recommending therapy before it has been scientifically proven to be effective in randomized controlled trials. This is not always practical to patients, though, since they wish to have therapy now."

Dr. Robert Clarke, from Radcliffe Infirmary in Oxford, England, adds,

> Elevated homocysteine levels due to deficiencies of folate and vitamin B_{12}, and perhaps other nutrients, are common in the elderly and appear to increase with age. These deficiencies are even more common in patients with dementia. It is unclear whether or not these elevated homocysteine levels are a cause or a consequence of having dementia. We believe that this hypothesis should be investigated further.

In my opinion, based on the knowledge we have thus far, the potential benefits of vitamin-B supplements for the elderly are probably greater than the potential risks. Most patients with early-onset AD are not willing to wait years for additional research to be published. If we wait too long, the condition of many patients could deteriorate to an irreversible stage.

In addition to the B vitamins, it is possible that methyl donors, such as TMG and SAMe, could be helpful.

Antioxidant Therapy

One of the first lessons I learned in pathology class my very first semester in medical school was that patients with Alzheimer's disease were afflicted with amyloidosis. Amyloidosis results from the deposit of protein fragments, called amyloid, around brain cells. Amyloid fragments join together to form small clumps, called amyloid fibrils. It is now fully accepted that the continued accumulation of amyloid leads to brain degeneration observed in Alzheimer's disease. Research indicates that amyloidosis may be a subsequence of inadequate antioxidant protection.

Neurons in the hypothalamus, an area of the brain involved in memory and learning, are particularly susceptible to oxidative damage in AD patients. Vitamin E is the best-studied antioxidant in terms of slowing down the progression of AD, but it's likely that quite a number of different antioxidants are also beneficial. A highly publicized article in the *New England Journal of Medicine* reported that the daily use of 1000 units of vitamin E was effective in slowing the progression of AD (Sano 1997). Researchers at the Rush Alzheimer's Disease Center, Rush University, in Chicago, Illinois, found through an epidemiological survey that the use of vitamin E and C supplements reduces the risk of developing AD (Morris 1998).

Several studies have examined the antioxidant capability of patients with AD. Researchers at the New York University Medical Center have discovered that there is a decrease in superoxide dismutase (SOD) and catalase antioxidant activity in neurons of patients with AD (Marcus 1998). SOD and catalase are natural antioxidants normally made within our bodies which protect our cells from damage.

Dr. De Deyn and colleagues, at the University of Antwerp in Belgium, analyzed the cerebrospinal fluid (CSF) of patients with AD, patients with Parkinson's disease, and healthy individuals, and came across some interesting findings (De Deyn 1998). The SOD activity in the CSF of patients with AD was significantly lower than that of the controls. However, SOD activity in patients with Parkinson's disease was no different than the controls. The researchers say, "The lowered SOD activity in Alzheimer's disease, as demonstrated here, may reflect impaired antioxidant defense mechanisms. Our findings should further motivate others to pursue antioxidant neuroprotective treatment strategies."

In the next chapter I will discuss a study that found a decrease in glutathione activity in brain cells of patients with Parkinson's disease. It appears that patients with PD have problems with the glutathione antioxidant defense system, while those with AD don't have enough antioxidant protection due to a shortage of SOD.

Melatonin, the sleep hormone, is known to have antioxidant activity. Researchers at the University of South Alabama College of Medicine, in Mobile, Alabama, report that melatonin inhibits the progressive formation of amyloid fibrils (Pappolla 1998); they say,

> Inhibition of fibrils could not be accomplished in control experiments when other antioxidants were substituted for melatonin under otherwise identical conditions. In sharp contrast with conventional antioxidants and available anti-amyloidogenic compounds, melatonin crosses the blood-brain barrier, is relatively devoid of toxicity, and constitutes a potential new therapeutic agent in Alzheimer's disease.

Providing Acetylcholine Precursors

There is a significant decline in levels of acetylcholine in patients with AD. Many approaches have been tried in order to elevate levels of this brain chemical. Studies providing precursors to acetylcholine such as choline, DMAE, CDP-choline, and lecithin, have not been successful to any large degree. For instance, fifty-one subjects with AD were given 20 grams a day of purified soy lecithin (containing 90 percent phosphatidylcholine) for six months (Little 1985). There were no differences between the placebo group and the lecithin group, but there was an improvement in a subgroup of relatively poor compliers, those who did not take the lecithin consistently.

CDP-choline is a compound that helps make phosphatidylcholine. When given to patients with AD at a daily dosage of 1000 mg orally for one month, it slightly improved mental performance (Cacabelos 1996). It would seem reasonable for patients with AD to take small amounts of choline, CDP-choline, lecithin, or a combination on a regular basis.

Improving Brain-Cell Membranes

Researchers from the Karolinska Institute in Huddinge, Sweden, have determined that the amount of polyunsaturated fatty acids present in the brain declines with age in AD patients (Soderberg 1991). Polyunsaturated fatty acids, such as DHA and arachidonic acid, which are normally found in the brain, were replaced by monounsaturated and saturated fatty acids. This change was not observed as clearly in the brains of patients who did not have AD.

Although the reason for these changes remains unclear, the researchers speculate that brain cells in AD patients lose the ability to effectively unsaturate fatty acids, and hence the cell membrane will end up with a preponderance of saturated and monounsaturated fatty acids. The loss of the long-chain polyunsaturated fatty acids, such as DHA, interferes with the proper function of the cell membrane. Dr. Soderberg and colleagues conclude, "The substantial decrease in polyunsaturated fatty acids may have serious consequences for cellular function. This could hamper the production of important active metabolites, such as prostaglandins and leukotrienes, which, in turn, could cause the changes observed in Alzheimer's disease."

A decline in polyunsaturated fatty acids, such as arachidonic acid and DHA, was also noticed by researchers at the University of Kentucky in Lexington (Prasad 1991). Perhaps damage to fatty acids by oxidation reduces the amount of long-chain polyunsaturated fatty acids in the brain. It seems reasonable, then, that therapy with polyunsaturated fatty acids, such as fish oils, may benefit patients with AD, especially when combined with antioxidants. However, no long-term studies are available to determine whether providing fish oils to patients with AD would lead to benefits.

In addition to treating patients with AD with fish oils and antioxidants, the use of phospholipids should be considered. However, it is not clear at this time whether therapy with lecithin or phosphatidylserine would provide long-term benefits.

Improving Energy Production

Enhancing the ability of brain cells to produce energy is certainly an additional option to consider. Several nutrients are available that are involved in neuronal metabolism.

A one-year-long study done in 1996 indicates that some patients with AD would benefit from supplementation with acetyl-L-carnitine. Lipoic acid and CoQ10 possibly could be helpful, but no formal studies have been published regarding their use in patients with AD.

Providing Anti-inflammatory Agents

Patients with AD have large amounts of neurofibrillary tangles in their brains. Neurofibrillary tangles result from the clumping of dead and damaged nerve cells. Many of these tangles contain a number of end products of inflammation. Studies have found that individuals who have used the nonsteroidal anti-inflammatory drugs (NSAIDs) aspirin, ibuprofen, and naproxen, have a reduced risk of AD. The use of acetaminophen is not associated with reduced risk.

NSAIDs have potentially serious risks and hence are not recommended as therapy for AD. We should keep in mind, though, that perhaps fish oils (or most omega-3 fatty acids) could be beneficial in reducing inflammation. The metabolites of these fatty acids have anti-inflammatory qualities not present in the fatty acid metabolites of omega-6 fatty acids. A low dosage of the common anti-inflammatory drug aspirin (i.e., 80 mg, a few times a week) should be considered.

Blocking the Breakdown of Acetylcholine

Another approach that has been tried in treating AD is to prevent the degradation of acetylcholine, the brain chemical associated with learning and memory. This can be achieved by providing drugs that block the activity of the enzyme cholinesterase, which breaks down acetylcholine. Two of these drugs are tacrine (Cognex) and donezepil (Aricept). Tacrine was first introduced in 1993, and donezepil in 1997. Although tacrine has shown modest benefits in treating Alzheimer's disease, it may induce liver damage.

A Chinese herbal extract called huperzine A has been shown in preliminary studies to block cholinesterase even more potently than tacrine (Xu 1995). Long-term studies with this herbal extract are not available.

Improving Blood Circulation

Any step taken to reduce atherosclerosis, or hardening of the arteries, is likely to improve blood circulation to the brain. A study in the *Journal of the American Medical Association* had good news about the herb ginkgo biloba (Le Bars 1997). Therapy with 40 mg of ginkgo three times a day for one year had a positive effect in patients with AD. There are several compounds in ginkgo that improve circulation and act as blood thinners and antioxidants.

Aspirin can also work as a blood thinner and improve circulation. Vinpocetine is another herbal extract that improves cerebral circulation.

Mood Improvement

Many patients with AD suffer from low mood or full-blown depression. Doctors sometimes prescribe Prozac and other serotonin reuptake inhibitors to these patients. It's possible that St. John's wort or other mood boosters, such as B vitamins or methyl donors, could be beneficial, although no formal testing has been done with these supplements and AD.

Combination Therapies

As I mentioned at the beginning of this chapter, we are not likely to find a magic nutrient or drug that, by itself, will treat AD adequately. The proper therapeutic approach to this disorder will come from the intelligent combination of different supplements and medicines. Only a few trials have been conducted using combination therapy.

In a study done by Biopharmaceutical Research Consultants in Ann Arbor, Michigan, lecithin, when added to tacrine, was found to provide a small additional benefit (Holford 1994). Lecithin was estimated to provide benefits equivalent to about 40 mg of tacrine. Women with AD who were already on estrogen replacement therapy were found to get additional cognitive benefits when tacrine was added to their regimen (Schneider 1997).

Eat Less, Think Longer

One additional approach to improving brain health is caloric restriction. Mark Mattson, Ph.D., Professor of Anatomy and Neurobiology at the University of Kentucky, says, "Our findings in animal studies show that eating less makes nerve cells in the brain more resistant to deterioration and death. This suggests that reduced calorie intake may help shield the brain, and could present a lifelong preventative strategy for neurodegenerative disorders such as Alzheimer's disease."

First-Line Therapy for AD

The nutritional approach to treating patients with AD is still very new, and no standards have been developed. It may take trial and error to find the ideal regimen for each patient. Here, I have provided a step-by-step guideline that you can review with your health-care practitioner and adapt to your particular situation.

- Therapy with the B vitamins should be the first approach. Use a B-complex that includes all the B vitamins, at about two to five times the RDA or PDV.
- Include plenty of fresh fruits and vegetables in order to obtain important carotenoids and flavonoids. Vitamin E, between 100 and 200 i.u. a day, preferably of mixed tocopherols, should be taken with a meal. You may recall that the *New England Journal of Medicine* study I mentioned earlier used 1000 units of vitamin E. My mind-boosting program recommends including many antioxidants in your regimen. Antioxidants help protect each other from being destroyed, so combining many antioxidants would reduce the dosage required for vitamin E. The dosage for vitamin C can range between 100 and 250 mg twice a day. A small dose of lipoic acid, such as 5 to 20 mg, is recommended.
- Fish oils supplying DHA and EPA, at 500 to 2000 mg a day, taken with meals, could well improve the composition of the cell membrane of neurons.

- Ginkgo biloba can sharpen thinking and improve memory. A 40-mg dose twice daily, with breakfast and lunch, is recommended. Ginkgo also provides antioxidant protection.
- Acetyl-L-carnitine is a nutrient that has shown promise in the therapy of AD. A dose of 100 to 250 mg before or with breakfast can be helpful in improving alertness and focus.
- CoQ10 at a dose of 30 mg with breakfast increases overall energy levels.
- Melatonin, in a dosage of 0.3 to 1 mg, one or two times a week, an hour or two before bed, can provide a deeper sleep in those who have mild insomnia.

Second-Line Therapy

The above suggestions should be helpful, but additional nutrients may be required. I recommend you next consider nutrients that have a direct influence on acetylcholine levels; these include choline, lecithin, DMAE, and CDP-choline. It is difficult to give precise dosages or combinations that would apply to all patients with AD. However, these proposed guidelines will help you and your health-care practitioner formulate the right program.

- Start with choline at 250 mg a day with breakfast or lunch. If choline itself is not effective, 100 mg of DMAE can be added. A new form of choline sold in health-food stores is CDP-choline. The dosage would be 100 to 250 mg in the morning. You may also consider adding about 1 gram of lecithin (phosphatidylcholine) a day, with breakfast or lunch. Please note that these four nutrients work in a similar manner, and their effects are cumulative. Consider taking a small amount of the methyl donors TMG or DMG, such as 50 to 100 mg, as a way to reduce homocysteine levels and provide more energy and improved mood.
- An exciting addition to the nutritional armamentarium of natural therapies for AD is the Chinese herbal extract known as huperzine A. Huperzine A works in a manner similar to the drug tac-

rine. It blocks the breakdown of acetylcholine in the brain, thus making more acetylcholine available to brain cells. A dosage of 0.02 to 0.05 mg per day can be tried instead of the standard cholinesterase inhibitors—*this must be done under medical supervision.* The dosage of huperzine A should be reduced if it is combined with nutrients that elevate acetylcholine levels, such as choline, DMAE, PC, and CDP-choline.

- Anti-inflammatory agents, such as ibuprofen and naproxen, have been shown in some studies to be beneficial, although the risks of stomach ulcers and kidney damage must be considered. Aspirin, at 80 mg a day, is a reasonable and safe amount to take as an anti-inflammatory agent—unless you are on anticoagulant therapy with coumadin or another blood-thinning agent.
- Some patients with AD have agitation or anxiety. The occasional use of kava or 5-HTP can be helpful in inducing relaxation. Vinpocetine is an herbal extract that improves circulation and could be considered in those who have poor circulation in the brain.

Cautions and Side Effects

Ginkgo, vinpocetine, fish oils, and aspirin are blood thinners; therefore, prudence is advised when they are combined, especially in high doses. Sometimes it is difficult to predict the reaction of a patient when multiple nutrients are used.

I recommend you constantly reevaluate the supplements being used. It's possible that with time, you may need fewer nutrients and smaller dosages, or just the opposite. The therapy of chronic diseases is a dynamic process, and adjustment of dosages is required on a regular basis.

Summary

Finding an effective therapy for AD is very challenging. However, with a great deal of patience, and trial and error, it is likely that a combination of nutrients can be found that can improve quality of life and cognitive function. Even though many nutritional options have been presented in this chapter, it is important not to take all of these supplements at the same time, but to gradually add one, and then another, in low doses, in order to determine the effectiveness of each nutrient. Sometimes you may build up tolerance to a particular nutrient, and you may need to substitute another. The use of nutrients is especially appropriate in thc treatment of AD since currently there is no effective pharmaceutical therapy for this condition.

TWENTY-TWO

Supplements for Patients with Parkinson's Disease

Parkinson's disease (PD) is a common neurological condition afflicting about 1 percent of men and women over the age of seventy. Individuals with PD have tremor of the hands, rigidity, poor balance, and mild intellectual deterioration. The tremor is most apparent at rest and is less severe with movement. In PD, a small region in the brain called the *substantia nigra* begins to deteriorate. The neurons of the substantia nigra use the brain chemical dopamine. With the loss of dopamine, tremors begin and movement slows. Despite current drug therapies, PD remains a progressive and incurable condition. Many patients with PD may also suffer from age-related cognitive decline or have some of the symptoms of Alzheimer's disease.

Although PD can occur from viral infections or exposure to environmental toxins, the causes of the majority of cases are not well known. Scientists suspect that oxidative damage to neurons in the substantia nigra could well be one of the major causes, particularly due to the depletion of the antioxidant glutathione (Pearce 1997).

TREATMENT STRATEGIES FOR PD

The nutritional therapy for Parkinson's disease is still uncharted territory. The most promising approach appears to be the use of antioxidants to slow the oxidation and damage to the substantia nigra. It's possible that additional nutritional approaches may be found in the future. In this chapter I have provided several options that you could consider under the supervision of a medical provider.

There are basically three types of drugs that are commonly prescribed for patients with PD. First, doctors prescribe dopamine precursors, such as L-dopa, which converts into dopamine. A second approach is using drugs that block the breakdown of dopamine. A common medicine used for this purpose is selegiline (also known as deprenyl). And third, drugs are provided that influence dopamine receptors directly. The two most commonly prescribed are bromocriptine and pergolide.

Over the past few decades, doctors have made important advances in the therapy of PD with pharmaceutical medicines. Yet several nutritional strategies exist which should be explored further.

Improving the Antioxidant System

Of all the nutritional strategies available to treat those with PD, antioxidants appear to be the most promising choices to prevent or slow the progression of this condition. Individuals whose diets include plenty of healthy foods containing antioxidants are less likely to develop PD. Patients should consume foods, such as fruits and vegetables, that contain glutathione or can help produce it. Cyanohydroxybutene, a chemical found in broccoli, cauliflower, brussels sprouts, and cabbage, is also thought to increase glutathione levels.

I recommend the following antioxidants to be taken in addition to standard pharmaceutical therapy.

- Vitamin E, between 100 and 400 international units a day, preferably of mixed tocopherols, taken with any meal.

- Vitamin C, between 100 and 250 mg twice a day. In addition to being an antioxidant, vitamin C also helps the production of L-dopa from tyrosine (Seitz 1998).
- Lipoic acid, 10 to 20 mg a day in the morning, with breakfast. LA is a powerful antioxidant and helps generate glutathione.
- N-acetyl-cysteine is an antioxidant that can help regenerate glutathione. A dose of 250 mg of NAC can be taken most mornings before breakfast. I don't recommend the daily use of NAC until more is known about this nutrient.
- Selenium is an antioxidant that can help increase levels of glutathione. A dose of 50 to 100 micrograms a day can be taken with any meal. Selenium is also normally found in over-the-counter multimineral pills.
- Melatonin is the sleep hormone with antioxidant abilities. A dose of 0.3 to 1 mg can be taken one or two hours before bed for those with occasional insomnia. Tolerance can develop with regular use, and since we don't know the long-term effects of nightly use, it's best to limit the frequency of use of melatonin to once or twice a week. In the 1980s, some individuals taking a synthetic drug called MPTP developed symptoms similar to Parkinson's disease. It was determined that MPTP causes an oxidative destruction of substantia nigra neurons. Interestingly, a study with rats has determined that the administration of melatonin is able to almost completely prevent the neurotoxicity from MPP, a toxin very similar to MPTP (Byung 1998). The rats on melatonin and MPP did not get symptoms of PD while the controls on MPP alone did. The researchers from Kyong Hee University in Seoul, Korea, say, "The present results support the hypothesis that melatonin may provide the useful therapeutic strategy for the treatment of oxidative stress-induced neurodegenerative disease such as PD."

Providing Dopamine Precursors

L-dopa, the immediate precursor to dopamine, is a nutrient available by prescription. L-dopa (often combined with carbidopa) is the most commonly used medicine to treat PD. It is possible that the use of L-dopa for prolonged periods causes oxidation and toxicity to brain cells. If this turns out to be true, it would further justify the recommendations that antioxidants be added to standard PD therapy. There is, as of yet, no clinical proof that taking antioxidant supplements help patients with PD live longer, but all indications point to the possibility that the course of the disease can be slowed by providing adequate antioxidant support.

Tyrosine is an amino acid that can be converted into L-dopa. But there is no reason to take tyrosine if L-dopa is available. Another way to increase dopamine levels is with the use of B vitamins, particularly NADH. Preliminary studies have shown some benefit with NADH in the therapy of PD. Although more research is needed, for the time being, it would seem reasonable to add NADH at a dose of 2.5 mg; NADH can be taken every other morning on an empty stomach. NADH may also help regenerate the antioxidant glutathione which could be beneficial. Be careful when you add NADH if you are already taking L-dopa or other medicines that treat PD, since the effects could be cumulative. The long-term effectiveness of NADH in patients with PD is currently not known. Taking between two to four times the RDA for the B vitamins seems to be a reasonable option.

Blocking Dopamine Breakdown

Dopamine is broken down in the brain by an enzyme called monoamine oxidase (MAO). When the activity of MAO is inhibited, dopamine stays around longer and this benefits those with PD. Several drugs are available that block the activity of MAO. Selegiline is the most effective and the one used most commonly. The prescribed dosage is 5 mg a day.

No nutrients are currently known that prevent the breakdown of dopamine. However, a study conducted on rats at the College of Humanities and Sciences, Beijing Union University, in Beijing, China, indicates that the Chinese herbs codonopsis and astragalus can inhibit MAO type B and increase the activity of the antioxidant SOD (Jin 1997). We don't have any human trials to determine whether these two herbs would benefit patients with PD. Although selegiline is a very helpful medicine, high doses may increase the risk of heart irregularities.

Additional Nutrients to Consider

The nutritional treatments for PD that I have recommended thus far include antioxidants, B vitamins, and NADH. There are additional options to consider. Some of these other nutrients may not be directly involved in making more dopamine, but could well improve general cognitive abilities. Many patients who have PD, especially the elderly, may have additional age-related cognitive decline. I would recommend waiting one or two weeks after starting a supplement before you add another one.

- Fish oils are recommended, at a dosage of 500 to 1000 mg a day of EPA/DHA, with meals. The role of fish oils in PD is not known, but they can generally improve overall brain health.
- Coenzyme Q10, at a dosage of 30 mg each morning, with breakfast. This nutrient improves the energy production in cells.
- Gingko biloba, at a dosage of 40 to 60 mg most days, with breakfast or lunch. This herb has antioxidant properties and helps improve memory and alertness.

Summary

It's quite likely that the proper use of natural supplements can reduce the necessary dosage of L-dopa, selegiline, and other drugs currently used to treat PD, or help slow the progression of the condition. There's still a great deal we need to learn about the nutritional treatment of PD.

GLOSSARY

ACETIC ACID—CH3COOH; a sour, colorless liquid found in vinegar.

ACETYL—CH3CO; a two carbon acetic acid molecule from which a hydroxyl group (OH) has been removed.

ACETYL-COENZYME A (ACETYL-COA)—a condensation product of acetic acid and coenzyme A. It is an intermediate in the transfer of two-carbon molecules in the metabolism of sugars and fatty acids.

ACETYLATION—the formation of an acetyl derivative.

ACETYLCHOLINE—a chemical formed by choline and an acetyl group. It is a neurotransmitter in the nervous system used to transmit nerve impulses. Acetylcholine slows down heart rate, dilates blood vessels, and increases activity of the gastrointestinal system. In the brain, acetylcholine is involved with learning and memory.

ACETYLCHOLINESTERASE—the enzyme that breaks down acetylcholine into choline and acetate or acetic acid. It is located in the synaptic cleft.

ACTH (ADRENOCORTICOTROPHIC HORMONE)—a hormone secreted by the pituitary gland. It stimulates the adrenal gland to make steroids, particularly cortisol. ACTH is released in response to stress, leading to high cortisol levels.

ADD (ATTENTION DEFICIT DISORDER)—a common neurological condition in children characterized by learning difficulties and poor attention.

ADHD (ATTENTION DEFICIT HYPERACTIVITY DISORDER)—similar to ADD; children with ADHD additionally suffer with poor impulse control and hyperactive behavior.

AFFECTIVE DISORDERS—psychological conditions involving mood, such as depression and bipolar disorder.

AGE-RELATED COGNITIVE DECLINE (ARCD)—the gradual loss of mental abilities with age.

AGONIST—a drug or compound capable of attaching to a receptor and initiating a reaction. Compare with antagonist.

ALKALOID—any of hundreds of compounds found in plants with a nitrogen atom connected to two carbon atoms, and often formed in a ring structure. Many commonly known chemicals and drugs are alkaloids, including nicotine, cocaine, quinine, morphine, and ephedrine.

ALZHEIMER'S DISEASE—A progressive brain disease leading to memory loss, interference with thinking abilities, and other losses of mental powers. Brain cells show degenerative damage. Neurons that use the neurotransmitter acetylcholine are most affected.

AMINO ACID—a molecule that contains nitrogen and serves as a unit of structure for proteins.

AMYLOID—any of a group of proteins that deposit in the brain and cause amyloidosis. Amyloidosis is often associated with Alzheimer's disease.

ANALGESIC—a drug that reduces or takes away pain.

ANDROGEN—a hormone that encourages the development of male sexual characteristics. Some of the androgens made by the adrenal glands are DHEA, androstenedione, and testosterone.

ANTAGONIST—a drug or compound that interferes with the action of, or counteracts the action of, another drug.

ANTIOXIDANT—a substance that combines with damaging molecules, neutralizes them, and thus prevents the deterioration of DNA, RNA, lipids, and proteins. Vitamins C, E, and beta-carotene are the best-known antioxidants, but more and more are being discovered each year.

ARCD—see Age-related cognitive decline.

ATHEROSCLEROSIS—a condition in which the arteries in the heart and other parts of the body accumulate plaque and become narrow, decreasing the flow of blood and increasing the risk for a clot; it's also known as "hardening of the arteries."

ATOM—the ultimate, indivisible, and smallest particle of an element. For instance, hydrogen and oxygen are atoms. When two hydrogen atoms and one oxygen atom get together, they form a molecule of water.

ATP (ADENOSINE TRIPHOSPHATE)—the primary energy currency of a cell, derived from the metabolism of glucose, amino acids, and fatty acids.

AYURVEDA—a traditional system of medicine practiced in India since the first century A.D. Ayurvedic practitioners combine herbs, oils, and other natural systems in treating diseases. Many herbs used in Ayurvedic medicine are now gaining popularity in Western countries.

BENZODIAZEPINE—a class of medicines such as Valium, Dalmane, and Xanax, that act on GABA receptors to induce relaxation and sleep. Too much, used too often, can lead to memory loss. There are also receptors in the brain for benzodiazepines.

BLOOD-BRAIN BARRIER—the filtering system that prevents some of the substances in the regular circulatory system to easily get into the brain. Most of the nutrient supplements discussed in this book have the ability to cross this barrier.

CAPILLARIES—very small, hairline-thin vessels supplying blood to tissues.

CARDIOLIPIN—one of the components of a cell membrane.

CATECHOLAMINES—neurotransmitters such as dopamine, norepinephrine, and epinephrine.

CATECHOLAMINERGIC SYSTEM—neurons that use catecholamines.

CELL—the smallest organized unit of living structure in the body. There are trillions of cells in humans. The brain alone has close to one trillion.

CELL MEMBRANE—a thin layer consisting mostly of fatty acids that surrounds each cell.

CENTRAL NERVOUS SYSTEM—the brain and the nerves in the spinal cord. The peripheral nervous system refers to the nerves in the body outside of the central nervous system.

CEREBRUM—the upper, main part of the brain, consisting of left and right sides. It controls voluntary thought and movements.

CEREBRAL CORTEX—the outer part of the cerebrum.

CHOLESTEROL—the most abundant steroid in animal tissues. It is present in some of the animal foods we eat. Our liver can also make some if there's not enough in our diet. Cholesterol is used to make steroid hormones.

CHOLINERGIC SYSTEM—brain cells that use the neurotransmitter acetylcholine.

COENZYME—a substance that is necessary or enhances the activity of an enzyme. Several vitamins act as coenzymes.

COGNITION—mental activities such as thinking, memory, perception, judgment, and learning.

COGNITIVE—involving cognition.

CONTROL—in any study, whenever a group of animals or humans are given a certain medicine, they are compared to a second group of animals or humans who are in similar circumstances regarding everything except the medicine. This second group is known as the control. This way, researchers can find out the role of the medicine independent of any other factors.

CORTISOL—same as hydrocortisone, a sterol (related to a steroid) secreted by the human adrenal glands. It is often released in high amounts during stress. High doses lead to interference with the proper functioning of the immune system.

COUMADIN—a drug that has blood-thinning abilities, often prescribed for patients who clot easily.

CROSSOVER—in a research study, the placebo and medicine groups are switched (crossed over) to determine a more accurate effect of the medicine. The group that initially got the medicine now gets the placebo, and the group that initially got the placebo now gets the medicine.

CYTOKINES—hormonelike small proteins secreted by the immune system.

CYTOPLASM—the fluid gel substance inside a cell, enclosed by the cell membrane. It does not include the nucleus.

DEMENTIA—the loss of intellectual function caused by a variety of disorders. Alzheimer's disease is a type of dementia.

DENDRITE—the treelike branching arms of a neuron.

DIOSGENIN—a saponin found in the roots of plants such as the yam. In the laboratory, parts of diosgenin can be cleaved in order to make certain steroids. Our body is not known to have the proper enzymes to convert diosgenin into pregnenolone, progesterone, or DHEA. Therefore, ingesting wild-yam extracts will not lead to DHEA production.

DOPAMINE—a neurotransmitter made from tyrosine and L-dopa.

DOPAMINERGIC—brain cells that use dopamine as their neurotransmitter.

DOUBLE-BLIND—a research study where neither the researchers nor the volunteers know who's getting the medicine and who's getting the placebo until the code is broken at the end of the study.

EPINEPHRINE—a hormone made by the medulla (center) of the adrenal gland, and also made in the brain and other parts of the nervous system. It is a potent stimulator of heart rate, tightens some blood vessels while relaxing others, and relaxes the bronchi (tubes) in the lungs. In the brain it is considered a neurotransmitter that leads to alertness and vigilance. Epinephrine is made from norepinephrine.

ESTROGEN—a hormone made by the ovaries, adrenal glands, and also in various cells of the body. Estrogen promotes female characteristics. The most common estrogens are estrone, estradiol, and estriol. Premarin, the product name of conjugated estrogens, is actually derived from the urine of horses.

EXCITOTOXIN—toxins that bind to certain receptors such as glutamate receptors in neurons, and cause injury or death to these neurons.

FAT—a greasy material found in animal tissues and made from glycerol attached to three fatty acids.

FATTY ACID—a long-chain molecule made of carbon atoms and capped at the end with a carboxyl group (COOH).

GABA—gamma-aminobutyric acid, a brain chemical that causes sedation. Medicines such as Valium act on receptors for GABA to induce relaxation. GABA also refers to the receptors themselves.

GLUCOCORTICOID—any steroidlike compound capable of significantly influencing some aspects of metabolism, such as the promotion of glycogen deposition in the liver, and having anti-inflammatory effects. Cortisol is the most potent of the naturally occurring glucocorticoids, but some synthetic derivatives, such as prednisone, are more potent.

GLUCOSE—a sugar found in foods, and the product of the digestion of starches. It is the primary compound metabolized for energy in the brain.

GLUTAMATE—an amino acid found in proteins that also acts as a neurotransmitter in the brain.

GLYCEROL—a three-carbon substance that forms the backbone of fatty acids in fats.

GONAD—a testicle or ovary.

HDL—see Lipoprotein.

HIPPOCAMPUS—a complex, convoluted structure located in the brain involved in many functions including memory.

HOMOCYSTEINE—an intermediary compound in the metabolism of the amino acid methionine. High levels in the blood can cause atherosclerosis. Recently it has been suspected that high amounts of homocysteine can also be toxic to neurons. B vitamins, particularly folic acid, B_{12}, and B_6, can lower homocysteine levels.

HORMONE—a chemical messenger produced by a gland or organ that influences a number of metabolic actions in nearby or distant cells.

HYDROGENATION—the process of adding hydrogen to unsaturated fatty acids in order to make them harder. Many processed foods are hydrogenated, making them potentially unhealthy.

HYPOTHALAMUS—a small area of the brain above and behind the roof of the mouth. The hypothalamus is prominently involved with the functions of the autonomic nervous system (the independent nervous system outside of voluntary control) and the hormonal system. It also plays a role in mood and motivation.

IMMUNE GLOBULINS—a group of proteins found in blood. Immune globlins (or immunoglobulins) fight off infections by attaching to and killing bacteria and viruses. The best known is gamma globulin.

IMMUNOMODULATORY—a substance that has an influence on the immune system.

IN VITRO—a Latin term, meaning a study performed in a laboratory and not involving animals or humans.

IN VIVO—a Latin term, meaning a study performed on animals or humans.

INOSITOL—an essential nutrient made from glucose that forms part of phosphatidylinositol, one of the phospholipids in the cell membrane. Inositol is widely available in foods and can be made in the human body when needed.

INSULIN—a hormone made by the pancreas that helps regulate blood-sugar levels.

INTERFERON—a small protein produced by white blood cells to fight some forms of cancer and infections, especially viral infections.

INTERLEUKIN—similar to interferon; a small protein produced by white blood cells to fight infections and some forms of cancer. There are many types of interleukins, numbered 1, 2, 3 . . . up to 10 or more. Some interleukins have beneficial effects, others are harmful.

LDL—see Lipoprotein.

LIBIDO—sex drive.

LIPID—a fat-soluble substance.

LIPOFUSCIN—"wear-and-tear" brown pigment granules consisting of lipid-containing residues of metabolism. These granules can be found in liver, brain, and heart muscle, and are a sign of aging.

LIPOPROTEINS—compounds that contain lipids and proteins. Almost all of the lipids in blood, including cholesterol, are transported as lipoprotein complexes. There are a number of these lipoproteins in blood. The two best known by the public are HDL (high density lipoproteins, the "good" cholesterol) and LDL (low density lipoproteins, the "bad" cholesterol).

LYMPHOCYTE—a type of white blood cell that fights infections. Two major types are B lymphocytes and T lymphocytes.

LYMPHOKINE—a substance released by lymphocytes to help with immune function. Interferon is a type of lymphokine.

MACROPHAGE—a large cell of the immune system that has the ability to be phagocytic, that is, engulf and kill germs. This cell is also thought to be involved in plaque formation in arteries.

MACULAR DEGENERATION—the macula is the small area in the retina of the eye, 3 to 5 millimeters in size, that provides the sharpest and clearest vision. The macula can degenerate with the aging process, perhaps due to oxidation. The fatty acid DHA is present in large amounts in the retina.

METABOLISM—the continuous chemical and physical processes in the body involving the creation and breakdown of molecules; for instance, glucose can be metabolized to release its energy as ATP.

METHYL—a molecule made of carbon and three hydrogen atoms. A methyl donor is any substance that can donate a methyl group to another molecule.

MITOCHONDRIA—the chemical factories of cells, where energy is made. Thousands of mitochondria are present in each cell.

MOLECULE—the smallest possible combination of atoms that retains the chemical properties of the substance. For instance, a molecule of water consist of three atoms—two are hydrogen and one is oxygen.

MONOAMINE OXIDASE—the enzyme that breaks down dopamine, norepinephrine, and epinephrine in synapses. Two types are present, types A and B. Certain drugs can inhibit the action of MAOs; these drugs are called MAO inhibitors.

MULTIPLE SCLEROSIS—a chronic disease in which there is loss of myelin (the covering of a nerve) in the central nervous system; it is characterized by speech defects and loss of muscular coordination.

NATURAL KILLER CELL—a type of white blood cell that can destroy certain cancer cells and germs.

NERVE-GROWTH FACTOR—a type of compound in the brain involved in stimulating the growth of nerve cells.

NEURAL—any structure composed of nerve cells.

NEURON—a cell in the brain. There are billions of neurons in the brain that communicate with each other, using neurotransmitters, through connections called synapses.

NEUROTRANSMITTER—a biochemical substance, such as norepinephrine, serotonin, dopamine, acetylcholine, and endorphin, that relays messages from one neuron to another.

NOREPINEPHRINE—a hormone made by the brain and the adrenal gland. It is similar in some ways to epinephrine, but weaker.

NSAID (NON-STEROIDAL ANTI-INFLAMMATORY DRUG)—a group of drugs, such as aspirin and ibuprofen, that reduce inflammation by acting on prostaglandins and other substances.

OMEGA—the twenty-fourth and final letter of the Greek alphabet. In naming fatty acids, omega signifies the last carbon on the chain.

OMEGA-3—fatty acids whose first double bond is three carbons away from the end.

OMEGA-6—fatty acids whose first double bond is six carbons away from the end.

ORGANELLE—a small structure in the cell. Mitochondria are a type of organelle.

OXIDANT—a substance that causes oxidation.

OXIDATION—the process by which a compound reacts with oxygen and loses a hydrogen or electron.

PDV (PERCENT DAILY VALUE)—a nutritional guideline on the appropriate doses of different vitamins and minerals required for good health. The values are similar to, but generally toward the upper range of, the RDA.

PEPTIDE—a compound made from two or more amino acids. Very long chains of amino acids are called proteins.

PERINATAL—occurring before, during, or after birth.

PEROXIDATION—the process by which fatty acids get oxidized.

PHOSPHOLIPIDS—fatty acids combined with the mineral phosphorus and other molecules that make up the lining of a cell membrane.

PLACEBO—a dummy pill that contains no active ingredient.

PLACEBO-CONTROLLED—a study where a group of volunteers gets a medicine and another group, called the control, gets a placebo.

PLATELET—a small, round, or oval cell found in the blood, which is involved in blood-clotting.

POSTPARTUM—the period after childbirth.

PRECURSOR—a substance that precedes, and is the source, of another substance; for instance, 5-HTP is the precursor to serotonin.

PRO-OXIDANT—a substance that causes oxidation and damage to cells and surrounding molecules. Some antioxidants in very high doses can turn into pro-oxidants.

PROSTAGLANDIN—one of a number of substances derived from fatty acids and involved in a number of important functions in tissues and cells.

RANDOMIZED—a study where the volunteers are assigned to receive a medicine or a placebo without bias.

RDA (RECOMMENDED DAILY ALLOWANCE)—a nutritional guideline proposed by the government on the appropriate doses of different vitamins and minerals required for good health. Some scientists think that ingesting more than the RDA for certain nutrients may provide additional health benefits. PDV, or percent daily value, is a number similar to the RDA.

RECEPTOR—a special arrangement on a cell that recognizes a molecule and interacts with it. This allows the molecule to either enter the cell or to stimulate it in a specific way. Neurotransmitters, such as serotonin, have receptors that they interact with.

REMETHYLATION—replacing a methyl group on a substance.

RETINA—the back of the eye where light falls and visual input is perceived and later transmitted to the brain for interpretation. The retina contains a large amount of the fatty acid DHA.

REUPTAKE—when a neurotransmitter is released into the synaptic cleft, it is either broken down by enzymes or returns back to the neuron that released it in the first place; the latter process is called a reuptake.

SAPONIN—compounds of plant origin found commonly in herbs such as ginseng, cat's claw, and licorice root, and some vegetables such as yams.

SEROTONERGIC—nerves that use serotonin for communication.

SEROTONIN—a brain chemical (neurotransmitter) that relays messages between brain cells (neurons). It is one of the primary mood-regulating neurotransmitters. It is derived from the amino acid tryptophan. Serotonin can also be converted to melatonin.

STEROID—a large family of chemical substances which includes hormones and drugs that have a chemical structure comprised of a few rings attached to each other. Most steroids contain twenty-seven or more carbon atoms.

STEROL—a steroid of twenty-seven or more carbon atoms with one OH (alcohol) group.

SUBSTANTIA NIGRA—a large, dark-colored cell mass in the middle of the brain involved in controlling movement. Damage to the SN leads to the movement disorder known as Parkinson's disease.

SYNAPSE—a connection between two neurons.

SYNAPTIC CLEFT—the small gap at a synapse, between neurons, where neurotransmitters are released.

TESTOSTERONE—a hormone made by the testicles and adrenal glands, and also in various cells of the body, that promotes masculine traits.

THROMBOXANE—a group of compounds biochemically related to the prostaglandins and initially made from fatty acids. Different fatty acids lead to different thromboxanes, and each type of thromboxane has a different action. For instance, thromboxane B-2 can induce clot formation.

TRANS-FATTY ACIDS—fatty acids that have been altered by food processing and take on abnormal shapes not normally useful to the body.

TRIGLYCERIDE—a type of fat that circulates in the bloodstream. A glycerol molecule forms the backbone to which one, two, or three fatty acids attach. High blood triglyceride levels can lead to atherosclerosis (blockage of arteries).

TRIPEPTIDE—a substance made from three amino acids.

BIBLIOGRAPHY

Baskys, A., and G. Remington. *Brain Mechanisms and Psychotropic Drugs.* CRC Press: Boca Raton, Florida, 1996.

Cass, H. *Natural Highs.*Tarcher/Putnam: New York, 2000.

Cooper, J. R.; Bloom, F. E.; and R. H. Roth. *The Biochemical Basis of Neuropharmacology.* Oxford University Press: New York, 1996.

Dean, W., Morgenthaler, J., and S. Fowkes. *Smart Drugs II: The Next Generation.* Health Freedom Publications: Menlo Park, California, 1993.

Frankel, P., and F. Madsen. *Stop Homocysteine Through the Methylation Process.* TRC Publications: Thousand Oaks, California 1998.

Lombard, J., and C. Germano. *The Brain Wellness Plan.* Kensington Press: New York, 1997.

Marks, D. B.; Marks, A.D.; and C. M. Smith. *Basic Medical Biochemistry: A Clinical Approach.* William and Wilkins: Baltimore, Maryland, 1996.

McKully, Kilmer. *The Homocysteine Revolution.* Keats Publishing: New Canaan, Connecticut, 1997.

Sahelian, Ray. *Creatine: Nature's Muscle Builder.* Avery Publishing Group: Garden City Park, New York, 1997; updated 1998.

Ibid. *DHEA: A Practical Guide.* Avery Publishing Group: Garden City Park, New York, 1996.

Ibid. *5-HTP: Nature's Serotonin Solution*. Avery Publishing Group: Garden City Park, New York, 1998.

Ibid. *Kava: The Miracle Antianxiety Herb*. St. Martin's Press: New York, 1998.

Schmidt, Michael. *Smart Fats: How Dietary Fats and Oils Affect Mental, Physical and Emotional Intelligence*. North Atlantic Books: Berkeley, California, 1997.

Seigel, G. W., Agranoff, B. W., Albers, R. W. and P. B. Molinoff, eds. *Basic Neurochemistry: Molecular, Cellular, and Medical Aspects*, 5th edition. Raven Press, Ltd.: New York, 1994.

Shils, M., Olson, J., and M. Shike, eds. *Modern Nutrition in Health and Disease*, 8th edition. Lea and Febiger: Philadelphia, 1994.

Simopoulos, A., and J. Robinson. *The Omega Plan*. HarperCollins: New York, 1998.

Stedman's Medical Dictionary, 26th edition. William and Wilkins: Baltimore, Maryland, 1995.

Teeguarden, Ron. *Radiant Health: The Ancient Wisdom of the Chinese Tonic Herbs*. Warner Books: New York, 1998.

Tyler, V. E. *The Honest Herbal*. Pharmaceutical Products Press: Binghamton, New York, 1993.

REFERENCES

Aloia, R., and W. Mlekusch, 1988. "Techniques of quantitative analysis of organ and membrane phospholipids and cholesterol." In *Methods of Studying Membrane Fluidity*. Alan R. Liss, Inc: New York.

Alvarez X. A., et al., 1997. "Citicoline improves memory performance in elderly subjects." *Methods Find. Exp. Clin. Pharmacol.* 19(3):201–10.

Babb, S. M., et al. 1996. "Differential effect of CDP-choline on brain cytosolic choline levels in younger and older subjects as measured by proton magnetic resonance spectroscopy." *Psychopharmacology* 127(2): 88–94.

Balestreri, R., et al., 1987. "A double-blind placebo-controlled evaluation of the safety and efficacy of vinpocetine in the treatment of patients with chronic vascular senile cerebral dysfunction." *J. Am. Geriatr. Soc.* 35(5):425–30.

Barak, A. J., et al., 1996. "Betaine, ethanol, and the liver: a review." *Alcohol* 13(4):395–8.

Barkworth, M. F., et al., 1985. "An early phase I study to determine the tolerance, safety and pharmacokinetics of idebenone following multiple oral doses." *Arzneimittelforschung* 35(11):1704–7.

Bell, K. M., et al., 1994. "S-adenosylmethionine blood levels in major depression: changes with drug treatment." *Acta. Neurol.Scand.* Suppl; 154:15–8.

Bella, R., et al., 1990. "Effect of acetyl-L-carnitine on geriatric patients suffering from dysthymic disorders." *Int. J. Clin. Pharmacol. Res.* 10(6): 355–60.

Benton, D., Griffiths, R., and J. Haller, 1997. "Thiamine supplementation on mood and cognitive functioning." *Psychopharmacology* (Berl). 129(1):66–71.

Benton, D., Haller, J., and J. Fordy, 1995. "Vitamin supplementation for one year improves mood." *Neuropsychobiology* 32(2):98–105.

Benton, D., and P. Y. Parker, 1998. "Breakfast, blood glucose, and cognition." *Am. J. Clin. Nutr.* 67(4):772S-778S.

Bergamasco, B., et al., 1994. "Idebenone, a new drug in the treatment of cognitive impairment in patients with dementia of the Alzheimer type." *Funct. Neurol.* 9(3):161–8.

Bertoni-Freddari, C., et al., 1991. "Neurobiology of the aging brain: morphological alterations at synaptic regions." *Arch. Geron. Ger.* 12: 253–60.

Bhattacharya, S. K., Satyan, K. S., and S. Ghosal, 1997. "Antioxidant activity of glycowithanolides from Withania somnifera." *Indian J. Exp. Biol.* 35(3):236–9.

Birdsall, T. C., 1998. "Therapeutic applications of taurine." *Altern. Med. Rev.* 3(2):128–36.

Birkmayer, G. D., et al., 1991. "The coenzyme nicotinamide adenine dinucleotide (NADH) as biological antidepressive agent: experience with 205 patients." *New Trends Clin. Neuropharm.* 5:75–86.

Birkmayer, J. G. D., et al., 1993. "NADH—a new therapeutic approach to Parkinson's disease, comparison of oral and parenteral application." *Acta Neurol. Scand.* 87(Suppl 146):32–35.

Birkmayer, J. G. D., et al., 1996. "The new therapeutic approach for improving dementia of the Alzheimer type." *Ann. Clin. Lab. Sci.* 26:1–9.

Black, J., et al., 1991. "Usual versus successful aging: some notes on experiential factors." *Neurobiol. Aging* 12:325–28.

Blanchard, J., et al., 1997. "Pharmacokinetic perspectives on megadoses of ascorbic acid. *Am. J. Clin. Nutr.* 66(5):1165–71.

Blokland, A., et al., 1999. "Cognition-enhancing properties of subchronic phosphatidylserine (PS) treatment in middle-aged rats: comparison of bovine cortex PS with egg PS and soybean PS." *Nutrition* 15(10):778–83.

Bottiglieri, T., Hyland, K., and E. H. Reynolds, 1994. "The clinical potential of S-adenosylmethionine in brain mapping, cerebrovascular hemodynamics, and immune factors." *Ann. N.Y. Acad. Sci.* 17;777: 399–403.

Bressa, G. M., 1994. "S-adenosyl-methionine (SAMe) as antidepressant: meta-analysis of clinical studies." *Acta. Neurol. Scand. Suppl.* 154:7–14.

Bruhwyler, J., et al., 1998. "Facilitatory effects of chronically administered citicoline on learning and memory processes in the dog." *Prog. Neuropsychopharmacol. Biol. Psychiatry* 22(1):115–28.

Busse, E., et al., 1992. "Influence of alpha-lipoic acid on intracellular glutathione in vitro and in vivo." *Arzneimitterlforschung* 42:829–31.

Byung, K., et al., 1998. "Melatonin protects nigral dopaminergic neurons from 1-methyl-4-phenylpyridinium (MPP) neurotoxicity in rats." *Neuroscience Letters* 245:61–64.

Cacabelos, R., et al., 1996. "Therapeutic effects of CDP-choline in Alzheimer's disease. Cognition, brain mapping, cerebrovascular hemodynamics, and immune factors." *Ann. N.Y. Acad. Sci.* 17;777:399–403.

Caffarra, P., et al., 1980. "The effect of Deanol on amnesic disorders. A preliminary trial (author's transl)." *Ateneo Parmense* [*Acta Biomed.*] 51(4):383–9.

Campbell, F., et al., 1998. "Placental membrane fatty acid-binding protein preferentially binds arachidonic and docosahexanoic acids." *Life Sciences* 63:235–40.

Cardoso, S. M., et al., 1998. "The protective effect of vitamin E, idebenone and reduced glutathione on free radical mediated injury in rat brain synaptosomes." *Biochem. Biophys. Res. Commun.* 29;246(3): 703–10.

Carta, A., et al., 1993. "Acetyl-L-carnitine and Alzheimer's disease: pharmacological considerations beyond the cholinergic sphere." *Ann. N.Y. Acad. Sci.* 4;695:324–6.

Caso Marasco, A. et al., 1996. "Double-blind study of a multivitamin complex supplemented with ginseng extract." *Drugs Exp. Clin. Res.* 22(6):323–9.

Cenacchi, T., et al., 1993. "Cognitive decline in the elderly: a double-blind, placebo-controlled multicenter study on efficacy of phosphatidylserine administration." *Aging: Clinical and Experimental Research* (Italy) 5:123–33.

Cestaro, B., 1994. "Effects of arginine, S-adenosylmethionine and polyamines on nerve regeneration." *Acta. Neurol. Scand.* Suppl; 154:32–41.

Charlton, C. G. 1997. "Depletion of nigrostriatal and forebrain tyrosine hydroxylase by S-adenosylmethionine: a model that may explain the occurrence of depression in Parkinson's disease." *Life Sciences* 61;5: 495–502.

Cheng, D. H., Ren, H., and X. C. Tang, 1996. "Huperzine A, a novel promising acetylcholinesterase inhibitor." *Neuroreport.* 20;8(1):97–101.

Cheng, D. H., and X. C. Tang, 1998. "Comparative studies of huperzine A, E2020, and tacrine on behavior and cholinesterase activities." *Pharmacol. Biochem. Behav.* 60(2):377–86.

Chung, H., et al., 1999. "Ginkgo biloba extract increases ocular blood flow velocity." *J Ocul. Pharmacol. Ther.* 15(3):233–40.

Cipolli, C., and G. Chiari, 1990. "Effects of L-acetylcarnitine on mental deterioration in the aged: initial results." *Clin. Ter. Mar.* 31;132 (6 Suppl):479–510.

Crook, et al., 1991. "Effects of phosphatidylserine in age-associated memory impairment." *Neurology* 41:644–49.

Crook, T., et al., 1992. "Effects of phosphatidylserine in Alzheimer's disease." *Psychopharmacology Bulletin* 28:61–66.

D'Angelo, L., et al., 1986. "A double-blind, placebo-controlled clinical study on the effect of a standardized ginseng extract on psychomotor performance in healthy volunteers." *J. Ethnopharmacol.* 16(1):15–22.

Davis, M. A., et al., 1993. "Differential effect of cyanohydroxybutene on glutathione synthesis in liver and pancreas of male rats." *Toxicol. Appl. Pharmacol.* 123:257–64.

Davis, S., et al., 1996. "Androgens and the postmenopausal woman." *J. Clin. Endocrinol. Metab.* 81:2759–63.

De Deyn, P. P., et al., 1998. "Superoxide dismutase activity in cerebrospinal fluid of patients with dementia and some other neurological disorders." *Alzheimer Dis. Assoc. Disord.* 12(1):26–32.

Dhuley, J. N., 1998. "Effect of ashwagandha on lipid peroxidation in stress-induced animals." *J. Ethnopharmacol.* 60(2):173–8.

Dini, A., et al., 1994. "Chemical composition of *Lepidium meyenii*." *Food Chemistry* 49: 347–49.

Drevon, C. A. 1992, "Marine oils and their effects." *Nutrition Reviews* 50(4):38–45.

Elsakka, M., et al., 1990. "New data referring to chemistry of *Withania somnifera* species." *Rev. Med. Chir. Soc. Med. Nat. Lasi.* 94(2):385–7.

Engel, R. R., et al., 1992. "Double-blind cross-over study of phosphatidylserine versus placebo in patients with early dementia of the Alzheimer type." *Eur. Neuropsychopharmacol.* 2(2):149–55.

Fariello, R. G., Ferraro, T. N., and G. T. Golden, 1988. "Systemic acetyl-L-carnitine elevates nigral levels of glutathione and GABA." *Life Sci.* 43:289–92.

Ferris, S. H., et al., 1977. "Senile dementia: treatment with deanol." *J. Am. Geriatr. Soc.* 25(6):241–4.

Fisman, M., et al., 1981. "Double-blind trial of 2-dimethylaminoethanol in Alzheimer's disease." *Am. J. Psychiatry* 138(7):970–2.

Flood, J., Morley, J., and E. Roberts, 1995. "Pregnenolone sulfate enhances post-training memory processes when injected in very low doses into limbic system structures: the amygdala is by far the most sensitive." *Proc. Natl. Acad. Sci.* 7;92:10806–10.

Forsyth, L. M., et al., 1998. "The use of NADH as a new therapeutic approach in chronic fatigue syndrome." Presented at the 1998 annual meeting of the American College of Allergy, Asthma and Immunology.

Gerster, H., 1998. "Can adults adequately convert alpha-linolenic acid (18:3n-3) to eicosapentaenoic acid (20:5n-3) and docosahexaenoic acid (22:6n-3)?" *Int. J. Vitam. Nutr. Res.* 68(3):159–73.

Gillin, J. C., et al., 1981. "Effects of lecithin on memory and plasma choline levels: a study in normal volunteers." In *Cholinergic mechanisms: phylogenetic aspects, central and peripheral synapses and clinical significance;* Pepeu, G., and Ladinsky, H., eds; New York: Plenum Press, 937–45.

Gillis, J. C., Benefield, P., and D. McTavish, 1994. "Idebenone. A review of its pharmacodynamic and pharmacokinetic properties, and therapeutic use in age-related cognitive disorders." *Drugs Aging* 5(2): 133–52.

Gispin, W., 1993. "Neuronal plasticity and function." *Clin. Neuropharm.* 16S:5–11.

Grioli, S., 1990. "Pyroglutamic acid improves the age-associated memory impairment." *Fundam. Clin. Pharmaco.* 4(2):169–73.

Hamazaki, T., et al., 1996. "The effect of docosahexanoic acid on aggression in young adults: a placebo-controlled double-blind study." *J. Clin. Invest.* 97;4:1129–1134.

Ibid., 1998. "Docosahexaenoic acid does not affect aggression of normal volunteers under nonstressful conditions. A randomized, placebo-controlled, double-blind study." *Lipids* 33(7):663–7.

Hansen, J. B., et al., 1998. "Effects of highly purified eicosapentanoic acid and docosahexaenoic acid on fatty acid absorption, incorporation into serum phospholipids and postprandial triglyceridemia." *Lipids* 33(2):131–8.

Hibbeln, J. R., 1998. "Fish consumption and major depression [letter]." *Lancet* Apr 18;351(9110):1213.

Hindmarch I., et al., 1991. "Efficacy and tolerance of vinpocetine in ambulant patients suffering from mild-to-moderate organic psychosyndromes." *Int. Clin. Psychopharmacol* 6(1):31–43.

Holford, N. H., and K. Peace, 1994. "The effect of tacrine and lecithin in Alzheimer's disease. A population pharmacodynamic analysis of five clinical trials." *Eur. J. Clin. Pharmacol.* 47(1):17–23.

Jin, Z., et al., 1997. "Anti-aging effects of codonopsis and astragalus combination." *International J. Oriental Med.* 22:57–63.

Joseph, J. A., et al., 1998. "Long-term dietary strawberry, spinach, or vitamin E supplementation retards the onset of age-related neuronal signal-transduction and cognitive behavioral deficits." *J. Neurosci.* 18(19):8047–55.

Jumpsen, J. A., et al., 1997. "During neuronal and glial cell development diet n-6 to n-3 fatty acid ratio alters the fatty acid composition of phosphatidylinositol and phosphatidylserine." *Biochimica et Biophysica Acta.* 1347:40–50.

Kalaria, R. N., and S. Harik, 1992. "Carnitine acetyltransferase activity in the human brain and its microvessels is decreased in Alzheimer's disease." *Ann. Neurol.* 32(4):583–6.

Kelly, G. S. 1997. "Clinical applications of N-acetylcysteine." *Altern. Med. Rev.* 3(2):114–27.

Ibid., 1997. "Pantethine: a review of its biochemistry and therapeutic applications." *Altern. Med. Rev.* 5:365–77. (Excellent review article.)

Kiss, B., and E. Karpati, 1996. "Mechanism of action of vinpocetine." *Acta. Pharm. Hung.* 66(5):213–24.

Klein, J., et al., 1998. "Regulation of free choline in rat brain: dietary and pharmacological manipulations." *Neurochem. Int.* 32(5–6): 479–85.

Labrie, F., et al., 1997. "Effect of 12-month dehydroepiandrosterone replacement therapy on bone, vagina, and endometrium in postmenopausal women." *J. Clin. Endocrinol. Metab.* 82:3498–3505.

Ladd, S. L., et al., 1993. "Effect of phosphatidylcholine on explicit memory." *Clinical Neuropharmacology* 16;6:540–9.

Landbo, C., and T. Almdal, 1998. ["Interaction between warfarin and coenzyme Q10."] *Ugeskr Laeger* 25;160(22):3226–7.

Laugharne, J. D., Mellor, J. E., and M. Peet, 1996. "Fatty acids and schizophrenia." *Lipids* 31 Suppl:S163–5.

Le Bars, P. L., et al., 1997. "A placebo-controlled, double-blind randomized trial of an extract of ginkgo biloba for dementia." *JAMA* 278:1327–32.

Linde, K, et al., 1996. "St. John's wort for depression—an overview and meta-analysis of randomized clinical trials." *British Medical Journal* 313: 253–8.

Little, A., et al., 1985. "A double-blind, placebo-controlled trial of high-dose lecithin in Alzheimer's disease." *Journal of Neurology, Neurosurgery & Psychiatry* 48(8): 736–42.

Loehrer, F. M., et al., 1997. "Influence of oral S-adenosylmethionine on plasma 5–methyltetrahydrofolate, S-adenosylhomocysteine, homocysteine and methionine in healthy humans." *Pharmacol. Exp. Ther.* 282(2):845–50.

Loehrer, F. M., et al., 1996. "Effect of methionine loading on 5–methyltetrahydrofolate, S-adenosyl-methionine and S-adenosylhomocysteine in plasma of healthy humans." *Clin. Sci.* (Colch) 91(1): 79–86.

Maccari, F., et al., 1990. "Levels of carnitines in brain and other tissues of rats of different ages: effect of acetyl-L-carnitine administration." *Experimental Gerontology* 25:127–34.

Marcus, D. L., et al., 1998. "Increased peroxidation and reduced antioxidant enzyme activity in Alzheimer's disease." *Exp. Neurol.* 150(1): 40–4.

Marsh, G. R., and M. Linnoila, 1979. "The effects of deanol on cognitive performance and electrophysiology in elderly humans." *Psychopharmacology* (Berl) 66(1):99–104.

McCaddon, A., and C. L. Kelly, 1994. "Familial Alzheimer's disease and vitamin B_{12} deficiency." *Age Ageing* 23(4):334–7.

McEwen, B. S., et al., 1997. "Ovarian steroids and the brain: implications for cognition and aging." *Neurology* 48(5 Suppl 7): S8–15.

Mehta, A. K., et al., 1991. "Pharmacological effects of *Withania somnifera* root extract on GABA receptor complex." *Indian J. Med. Res.* 94: 312–5.

Mohs, R. C., et al., 1980. "Choline chloride effects on memory in the elderly." *Neurobiol. Aging* 1:21–5.

Morcos, N. C., 1997. "Modulation of lipid profile by fish oil and garlic combination." *J. Natl. Med. Assoc.* 89(10):673–8.

Mordente, A., et al., 1998. "Antioxidant properties of 2,3-dimethoxy-5-methyl-6-(10-hydroxydecyl)-1,4-benzoquinone (idebenone). *Chem. Res. Toxicol.* 11(1):54–63.

Morris, M. C., et al., 1998. "Vitamin E and vitamin C supplement use and risk of incident Alzheimer disease." *Alzheimer. Dis. Assoc. Disord.* 12(3):121–6.

Orvisky, E., et al., 1997. "High-molecular-weight hyaluronan—a valuable tool in testing the antioxidative activity of amphiphilic drugs stobadine and vinpocetine" *J. Pharm. Biomed. Anal.* 16(3):419–24.

Ortega, R. M., et al., 1997. "Dietary intake and cognitive function in a group of elderly people." *Am. J. Clin. Nutr.* 66(4):803–9.

Packer, L., Roy, S., and C. K. Sen, 1997. "Alpha-lipoic acid: a metabolic antioxidant and potential redox modulator of transcription." *Advances in Pharmacology* 38: 79–101.

Pappolla, M., et al., 1998. "Inhibition of Alzheimer beta-fibrillogenesis by melatonin." *J. Biol. Chem. Mar.* 27;273(13):7185–8.

Parnetti, L., 1995. "Clinical pharmacokinetics of drugs for Alzheimer's disease." *Clin. Pharmacokinet.* 29(2):110–29.

Parnetti, L., Bottiglieri, T., and D. Lowenthal, 1997. "Role of homocysteine in age-related vascular and non-vascular diseases." *Aging* (Milano) 9(4):241–57.

Passeri, M., et al., 1990. "Acetyl-L-carnitine in the treatment of mildly demented elderly patients." *Int. J. Clin. Pharmacol. Res.* 10(1–2):75–9.

Pearce, R. K., et al., 1997. "Alterations in the distribution of glutathione in the substantia nigra in Parkinson's disease." *J. Neural Transm.* 104(6–7):661–77.

Peet, M., et al., 1998. "Depletion of omega-3 fatty acid levels in red blood cell membranes of depressive patients." *Biol. Psychiatry* 1;43(5): 315–9.

Perkins, A. et al., 1999. "Association of antioxidants with memory in a multiethnic elderly sample using the third national health and nutrition examination survey." *Am. J. Epid.* 150:37–44.

Pettegrew, J., et al., 1995. "Clinical and neurochemical effects of acetyl-L-carnitine in Alzheimer's disease." *Neurobiology of Aging* 16;1:1–4.

Piovesan, P., et al., 1994. "Acetyl-L-carnitine treatment increases choline acetyltransferase activity and NGF levels in the CNS of adult rats following total fimbria-fornix transection." *Brain Research*. 633: 77–82.

Pisano, P., et al., 1996. "Plasma concentrations and pharmacokinetics of idebenone and its metabolites following single and repeated doses in young patients with mitochondrial encephalomyopathy." *Eur. J. Clin. Pharmacol.* 51(2):167–9.

Porciatti V, et al., 1998. "Cytidine-5'-diphosphocholine improves visual acuity, contrast sensitivity and visually-evoked potentials of amblyopic subjects." *Curr. Eye. Res.* 17(2):141–8.

Prasad, M. R., et al., 1991. "Regional membrane phospholipid alterations in Alzheimer's disease." *Neurochemical Research* 23(1):81–88.

Purmova, J., and L. Opletal, 1995. "Phytotherapeutic aspects of diseases of the cardiovascular system. Saponins and possibilities of their use in prevention and therapy." *Ceska. Slov. Farm.* 44(5):246–51.

Qian, B. C., et al., 1995. "Pharmacokinetics of tablet huperzine A in six volunteers." *Chung Kuo Yao Li Hsueh Pao* 16(5):396–8.

Rai, G., et al., 1990. "Double-blind, placebo-controlled study of acetyl-L-carnitine in patients with Alzheimer's dementia." *Curr. Med. Res. Opin.* 11(10):638–47.

Refsum, H., et al., 1998. "Homocysteine and cardiovascular disease." *Annu. Rev. Med.* 49:31–62.

Riggs, K. M., et al., 1996. "Relations of vitamin B_{12}, vitamin B_6, folate, and homocysteine to cognitive performance in the normative aging." *Am. J. Clin. Nutr.* 63(3):306–14.

Sahelian, R., and S. Borken, 1998. "DHEA and cardiac arrhythmia." *Ann. Int. Med.* Oct 1; volume 129;7:588.

Rupprecht, R., and F. Holsboer, 1999. "Neuroactive steroids: mechanisms of action and neuropsychopharmacological perspectives." *Trends Neurosci.* 22(9):410–6.

Salmaggi, P., et al., 1993. "Double-blind, placebo-controlled study of S-adenosyl-L-methionine in depressed postmenopausal women." *Psychother. Psychosom.* 59(1):34–40.

Sano, M., et al., 1997. "A controlled trial of selegiline, alpha-tocopherol, or both as treatment for Alzheimer's disease." *N. Engl. J. Med.* 336: 1216–22.

Schliebs, R., 1997. "Systemic administration of defined extracts from *Withania somnifera* (Indian ginseng) and Shilajit differentially affects cholinergic but not glutamatergic and GABAergic markers in rat brain." *Neurochem. Int.* 30(2):181–90.

Schneider, L. S., and M. Farlow, 1997. "Combined tacrine and estrogen replacement therapy in patients with Alzheimer's disease." *Ann. N.Y. Acad. Sci.* 26;826:317–22.

Schoenen, J., et al., 1998. "Effectiveness of high-dose riboflavin in migraine prophylaxis. A randomized controlled trial." *Neurology* 50(2): 466–70.

Secades, J. J., and G. Frontera, 1995. "CDP-choline: pharmacological and clinical review. *Methods Find Exp. Clin. Pharmacol.* 17 Suppl B:2–54.

Seitz, G., et al., 1998. "Ascorbic acid stimulates DOPA synthesis and tyrosine hydroxylase gene expression in the human neuroblastoma cell line SK-N-SH." *Neuroscience Letters* 244:33–36.

Sergio, W., 1988. "Use of DMAE (2–dimethylaminoethanol) in the induction of lucid dreams." *Med. Hypotheses* 26(4):255–7.

Shigenaga, M. K., et al., 1994. "Oxidative damage and mitochondrial decay in aging." *Proc. Natl. Acad. Sci.* 8;91(23):10771–8.

Shults, C. W., et al., 1998. "Absorption, tolerability, and effects on mitochondrial activity of oral coenzyme Q10 in parkinsonian patients." *Neurology.* 50(3):793–5.

Shults, C. W., et al., 1997. "Coenzyme Q10 levels correlate with the activities of complexes I and II/III in mitochondria from Parkinsonian and nonParkinsonian subjects." *Ann. Neurol.* 42(2):261–4.

Singh, H. K., and B. N. Dhawan, 1982. "Effect of *Bacopa monniera Linn.* (brahmi) extract on avoidance responses in rat." *J. Ethnopharmacol.* 5(2):205–14.

Sitaran, N., Weingartner, H., and J. C. Gillin, 1978. "Human serial learning: enhancement with arecholine and choline and impairment with scopolamine." *Science* 201:274–6.

Skaper, S. D., et al., 1998. "Melatonin prevents the delayed death of hippocampal neurons induced by enhanced excitatory neurotransmission and the nitridergic pathway." *FASEB J.* 12(9):725–31.

Skolnick, A. A., 1997. "Old Chinese herbal medicine used for fever yields possible new Alzheimer disease therapy [news]." *JAMA.* 12; 277(10):776.

Soderberg, M., et al., 1991. "Fatty acid composition of brain phospholipids in aging and in Alzheimer's disease." *Lipids* 26:421–5.

Sorgatz, H., 1987. "Effects of lecithin on memory and learning." In *Lecithin: technological, biological, and therapeutic aspects.* Hanin, I., Ansell, G. G., eds.; Proceedings of the fourth international colloquium on lecithin. New York: Plenum Press: 147–53.

Sotaniemi, E. A., et al., 1995. "Ginseng therapy in non-insulin-dependent diabetic patients." *Diabetes Care* 18(10):1373–5.

Spagnoli, A., et al., 1991. "Long-term acetyl-L-carnitine treatment in Alzheimer's disease." *Neurology* 41(11):1726–32.

Spallholz, J. E., 1997. "Free radical generation by selenium compounds and their pro-oxidant toxicity." *Biomed. Environ. Sci.* 10(2–3):260–70.

Sprong, R. C., et al., 1998. "Low-dose N-acetylcysteine protects rats against endotoxin-mediated oxidative stress, but high-dose increases mortality." *Am. J. Respir. Crit. Care Med.* 157(4 Pt 1):1283–93.

Stoll, S., et al., 1993. "The potent free radical scavenger alpha-lipoic acid improves memory in aged mice. Putative relationship to NMDA receptor deficits." *Pharmacol. Behav.* 46: 799–805.

Stoll, A. L., et al., 1996. "Choline in the treatment of rapid-cycling bipolar disorder; clinical and neurochemical findings in lithium-treated patients." *Biol. Psychiatry* 40(5):382–8.

Strijks, E., Kremer, H. P., and M. W. Horstink, 1997. "CoQ10 therapy in patients with idiopathic Parkinson's disease." *Mol. Aspects Med.* 18 Suppl:S237–40.

Subhan, Z., 1985. "Psychopharmacological effects of vinpocetine in normal healthy volunteers." *Eur. J. Clin. Pharmacol.* 28(5):567–71.

Suzuki, H., et al., 1998. "Effect of the long-term feeding of dietary lipids on the learning ability, fatty acid composition of brain stem phospholipids and synaptic membrane fluidity in adult mice: a comparison of sardine oil diet with palm oil diet." *Mechanisms of Ageing and Development* 101: 119–28.

Suzuki, K., 1981. "Chemistry and metabolism of brain lipids." In *Basic Neurochemisty*, 3rd edition; Seigel, G.J., et al., eds., Little, Brown: Boston, 355–70.

Teri, L., McCurry, S., and R. Logsdon, 1997. "Memory, thinking, and aging. What we know about what we know." *West. J. Med.* 167: 269–75.

Thal, L. J., et al., 1989. "The safety and lack of efficacy of vinpocetine in Alzheimer's disease." *J. Am. Geriatr. Soc.* 37(6):515–20.

Thal, L. J., et al., 1996. "A 1-year multicenter placebo-controlled study of acetyl-L-carnitine in patients with Alzheimer's disease." *Neurology* 47:705–11.

Tripathi, Y. B., et al., 1996. "*Bacopa monniera Linn* as an antioxidant: mechanism of action." *Indian J. Exp. Biol.* 34(6):523–6.

Tweedy, J. R., and C. A. Garcia, 1982. "Lecithin treatment of cognitively impaired Parkinson's patients." *Eur. J. Clin. Invest.* 12(1):87–90.

Uchida, K., 1998. "Induction of apoptosis by phosphatidylserine." *J. Biochem.* (Tokyo) 123(6):1073–8.

Urban, T., et al., 1997. "Neutrophil function and glutathione-peroxidase activity in healthy individuals after treatment with N-acetyl-L-cysteine." *Biomed. Pharmacother.* 51:388–90.

Villanueva, L., et al., 1991. "Depressive effects of mu and delta opioid receptor agonists on activities of dorsal horn neurons are enhanced by dibencozide." *J. Pharmacol. Exp. Ther.* 257(3):1198–202.

Volz, H. P., and M. Kieser, 1997. "Kava-kava extract WS 1490 versus placebo in anxiety disorders—a randomized placebo-controlled 25-week outpatient trial." *Pharmacopsychiatry* 30:1–5.

Vrecko, K., et al., 1997. "NADH stimulates endogenous dopamine biosynthesis by enhancing the recycling of tetrahydrobiopterin in rat pheochromocytoma cells." *Biochimica et Biophysica Acta* 1361: 59–65.

Wakabayashi, C., et al., 1998. "An intestinal bacterial metabolite of ginseng protopanaxadiol saponins has the ability to induce apoptosis in tumor cells." *Biochem. Biophys. Res. Comm.* 246:725–30.

Westermarck, T., 1997. "Evaluation of the possible role of coenzyme Q10 and vitamin E in juvenile neuronal ceroid-lipofuscinosis (JNCL)." *Mol. Aspects Med.* 18 Suppl:S259–62.

Weyer, G., et al., 1997. "A controlled study of 2 doses of idebenone in the treatment of Alzheimer's disease." *Neuropsychobiology* 36(2):73–82.

Wesnes, K. A., et al., 1997. "The cognitive, subjective, and physical effects of a ginkgo biloba/panax ginseng combination in healthy volunteers with neurasthenic complaints." *Psychopharmacol. Bull.* (4):677–83.

Wiebke, A., et al., 1999. "Dehydroepiandrosterone replacement in women with adrenal insufficiency." *N. Engl. J. Med.* 341:1013–20.

Wilkinson, T. J., et al., 1997. "The response to treatment of subclinical thiamine deficiency in the elderly." *Am. J. Clin. Nutr.* 66(4):925–8.

Williams, C. L., et al., 1998. "Hypertrophy of basal forebrain neurons and enhanced visuospatial memory in perinatally choline-supplemented rats." *Brain Res.* 1;794(2):225–38.

Wood, J. L., and R. G. Allison, 1982. "Effects of consumption of choline and lecithin on neurological and cardiovascular systems." *Fed. Proc.* 41(14):3015–21.

Woodside, J. V., et al., 1998. "Effect of B-group vitamins and antioxidant vitamins on hyperhomocysteinemia: a double-blind, randomized, factorial-design, controlled trial." *Am. J. Clin. Nutr.* 67(5):858–66.

Wurtman, R. J., 1992. "Choline metabolism as a basis for the selective vulnerability of cholinergic neurons." *Trends in Neurosci.* 15:117–22.

Xu, S. S., et al., 1995. "Efficacy of oral huperzine-A on memory, cognition, and behavior in Alzheimer's disease." *Chung Kuo Yao Li Hsueh Pao* 16(5):391–5.

Yaffe, K., et al., 1998. "Estrogen therapy in postmenopausal women: effects on cognitive function and dementia." *JAMA* 279:688–95.

Yamada, K., et al., 1997. "Orally active NGF synthesis stimulators: potential therapeutic agents in Alzheimer's disease." *Behav. Brain Res.* 83(1–2):117–22.

Yehuda, S., et al., 1998. "Modulation of learning and neuronal membrane composition in the rat by essential fatty acid preparation: time-course analysis." *Neurochem. Res.* 23(5):627–34.

Yen, S. S., Morales, A. J., and O. Khorram, 1995. "Replacement of DHEA in aging men and women." *Ann. NY. Acad. Sci.* 774:128–42.

Zeisel, S. H. 1997. "Choline: essential for brain development and function." *Adv. Pediatr.* 44:263–95.

Zeisel, S. H., and J. K. Blusztajn, 1994. "Choline and human nutrition." *Annu. Rev. Nutr.* 14:269–96.

Zeisel, S. H., et al., 1991. "Choline, an essential nutrient for humans." *FASEB J.* 5, 2093–98.

Zeisel, S. H., et al., 1980. "Normal plasma choline responses to ingested lecithin." *Neurology* 30(11):1226–29.

Zhang, R. W., et al., 1991. "Drug evaluation of huperzine A in the treatment of senile memory disorders." *Chung Kuo Yao Li Hsueh Pao.* 12(3):250–2.

Zhao, X. Z., et al., 1990. "Antisenility effect of ginseng-rhizome saponin." *Chung Hsi I Chieh Ho Tsa Chih* 10(10):586–9, 579.

Zumoff, B., et al., 1996. "Twenty-four-hour mean plasma testosterone concentration declines with age in normal premenopausal women." *J. Clin. Endocrinol. Metab.* 80:1429–30.

INDEX

Note: The principal page references to a topic are in *italics*.